Clinical Record Book

for

Adult Health Nursing - I

Clinical Record Book for **Adult Health Nursing - I**

As per the Revised Nursing Syllabus

Dipak Sethi PhD
Dean and Professor
Noida International University
College of Nursing
Greater Noida, Uttar Pradesh, India

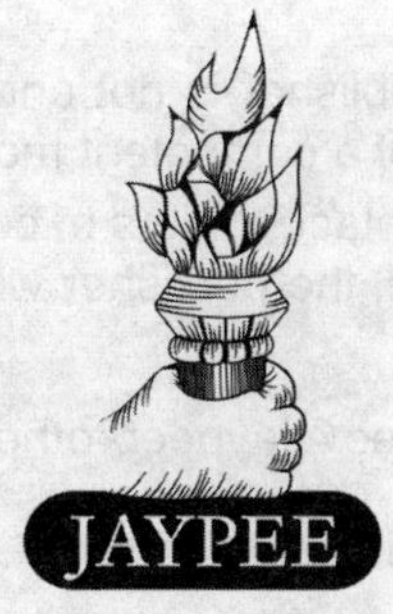

JAYPEE BROTHERS MEDICAL PUBLISHERS
The Health Sciences Publisher
New Delhi | London

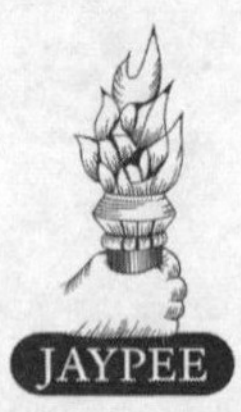

Jaypee Brothers Medical Publishers (P) Ltd

Headquarters
EMCA House
23/23-B, Ansari Road, Daryaganj
New Delhi 110 002, India
Landline: +91-11-23272143, +91-11-23272703
+91-11-23282021, +91-11-23245672
E-mail: jaypee@jaypeebrothers.com

Corporate Office
Jaypee Brothers Medical Publishers (P) Ltd.
4838/24, Ansari Road, Daryaganj
New Delhi 110 002, India
Phone: +91-11-43574357
Fax: +91-11-43574314
E-mail: jaypee@jaypeebrothers.com

Overseas Office
JP Medical Ltd.
83, Victoria Street, London
SW1H 0HW (UK)
Phone: +44-20 3170 8910
E-mail: info@jpmedpub.com

EU GPSR Authorised Representative
Logos Europe, 9 rue Nicolas Poussin
17000, La Rochelle, France
Phone: +33 (0) 6 67 93 73 78
E-mail: Contact@logoseurope.eu

Website: www.jaypeebrothers.com
Website: www.jaypeedigital.com

Inquiries for bulk sales may be solicited at: jaypee@jaypeebrothers.com

Clinical Record Book for Adult Health Nursing - I

First Edition: 2024

Revised Reprint: 2024, 2025, 2026

ISBN: 978-93-5696-832-5

Printed in India by K.K. Printers, Kundli, Haryana-131 028.

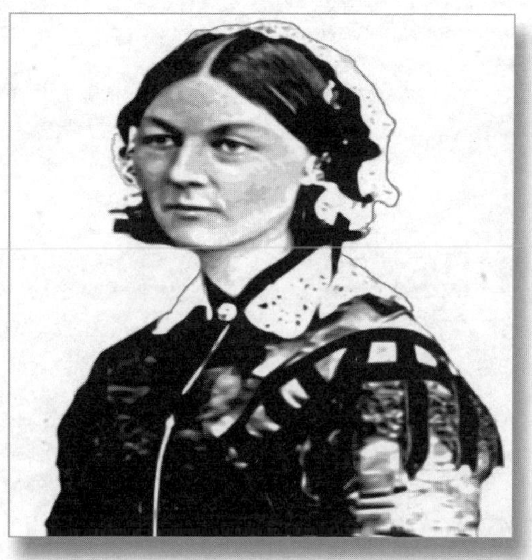

Pledge

I solemnly pledge in the presence of this assembly
To render nursing services with due respect
For the dignity and rights of the people I serve
I will, at all times, respect the values and beliefs
Of the people entrusted to my care
And will make no distinction of caste, creed or race
In the performance of my duties
I will strive in the practice of my profession
To promote health, prevent illness, alleviate sufferings,
And restore health of the people I serve
I will hold in trust personal information
Of a confidential nature
And use my best judgment in sharing this
With responsible persons
I will strive to maintain co-operative relationship
With fellow-workers in nursing and other fields
I will try to maintain standard of personal conduct
That will reflect credit upon my profession.
I will strive to observe the code of nursing ethics
As laid down by my profession.

Source: Nightingale Pledge and Code for Nurses 1973.

Preface

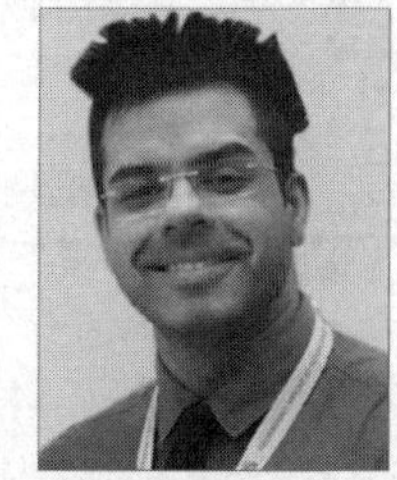

The healthcare sector is evolving to accommodate the prevailing demands of society. With the expansion of nursing education, the responsibilities of nursing students are also undergoing significant changes. The students in this period of tremendous change in the healthcare delivery system need a set of beliefs and skills. In order to adapt these developments, I have undertaken an attempt to create a clinical record book for Adult Health Nursing. This clinical activity record book for BSc Nursing degree is drafted as per the revised nursing syllabus. The objective is to standardize the curriculum in order to have a consistent structure throughout all nursing institutions. Nursing is a career that requires nurses to possess a comprehensive understanding of three educational domains—cognitive, psychomotor, and communication skills. The psychomotor domain refers to the ability to perform different nursing procedures. Adequate information, perfection in executing skills and procedures, and repeated practice are essential components of clinical practice. The clinical activities documented in this record book are the essential prerequisites for obtaining a BSc degree. The primary objectives of clinical experience include the student's ability to apply theoretical information in practical settings, as well as acquire a range of nursing skills based on scientific principles.

Dipak Sethi

Student Profile

Paste your passport size photo

Name of the Student: ....

PRN No.: ....

Batch: ....

Name of the Institute: ....

Signature of Student

Signature of Subject In-Charge

Signature of Principal

Adult Health Nursing

CLINICAL REQUIREMENTS

S. no.	Contents	Maximum Marks	Marks Obtained	Signature of the Teacher
I.	**Nursing Care Plan on Medical Disorders:** ◆ Care Plan/Care Study ◆ Health Education ◆ Clinical Presentation/Care Note			
II.	**Nursing Care Plan Surgical Conditions:** ◆ Care Plan/Care Study ◆ Health Education ◆ Clinical Presentation			
III.	**Nursing Care Plan Cardiac Disorders:** ◆ Care Plan/Care Study ◆ Clinical Presentation ◆ Cardiac Assessment ◆ Drug Presentation			
IV.	**Nursing Care Plan on Communicable Disease:** ◆ Care Plan/Care Study ◆ Case Presentation/Care Note			
V.	**Nursing Care Plan on Musculoskeletal System Disorder:** ◆ Care Plan/Care Study ◆ Case Presentation/Care Note			
VI.	**Nursing Management of Patients in the Operating Rooms** **Assist as a Scrub Nurse in Major Operation Theater:** 1. 2. 3. 4.			

S. no.	Contents	Maximum Marks	Marks Obtained	Signature of the Teacher
VII.	**Assist as a Scrub Nurse in Minor Operation Theater:** 1. 2. 3. 4.			
VIII.	**Positioning and Draping:** 1. 2. 3. 4. 5.			
IX.	**Assist as Circulatory Nurse:** 1. 2. 3. 4.			

____

Signature of the Internal Examiner

Name: ....

Date: ....

____

Signature of the External Examiner

Name: ....

Date: ....

Supplementary Examination

____

Signature of the Internal Examiner

Name: ....

Date: ....

____

Signature of the External Examiner

Name: ....

Date: ....

Contents

Care Plan

Evaluation Criteria for Nursing Care Plan – 1

S. No.	Contents	Maximum marks	Allotted marks
1.	Patient's History	02	
2.	Physical Examination	02	
3.	Investigations	01	
4.	Drug Study	02	
5.	Nursing Care Plan		
	◆ Assessment	02	
	◆ Nursing Diagnosis	02	
	◆ Goals	01	
	◆ Expected Outcome	01	
	◆ Nursing Intervention	03	
	◆ Rationale	01	
	◆ Evaluation	02	
6.	Nurses' Notes	03	
7.	Health Education	02	
8.	Bibliography	01	
	Total	**25**	

Remarks:

Signature of Student

Signature of Supervisor

NURSING CARE PLAN – 1

Patient's Identification Data

- Name:
- Age:
- Sex:
- Marital status:
- Hospital registration no.:
- Ward/bed no.:
- Address:
- Tel. no.:
- Religion:
- Education:
- Date of admission:
- Date of discharge:
- Diagnosis:
- Operation:
- Date of operation:
- Name of the doctor:
- Occupation:
- Monthly family income (₹):
- Nursing alert:
- Sensitivity/allergy/precaution:
- Weight:
- Height:

Chief Complaints with Duration

History of Present Illness

History of Past Medical Illness: Illness/medications/any restrictions

History of Past Surgical Illness: Illness/medications/any restrictions

Obstetrical History

No. of pregnancy	Year	Type of delivery	Gender of baby	Puerperium	Remarks

Family History

S. No.	Name of family member	Age and gender	Relationship with patient	Occupation	Health status/H/o significant illness	Health habits

Family Tree

Genogram key:

Female = ○

Male = □

Patient = Point to Patient ↗

Deceased = ■ or ●

( ) = Cause of death

⋮ = Adoption (vertical)

Consanguinity = □═○

Socioeconomic History

- Occupation and social relationship
- Monthly family income
- Health facility near home: Hospital/health center/any other: If any other (specify)

Transportation Facility

Yes/No

Housing

Type: Kutcha/Pucca

- Number of rooms
- Toilet: Indian/western/temporary/open
- Electricity: Yes/No
- Drinking water source: Tap/well/pond/river/hand/pump

Dietary History

Health Habits: Functional Health Pattern

- Health perception/health management:
- Nutritional/metabolic:
- Elimination:
- Activity/exercise:
- Sleep/rest:
- Self-perception/self-concept:
- Role relationship:
- Sexuality/reproductive:
- Coping/stress-tolerance:
- Value/belief:
- Other comments/data:

Physical Examination

General Appearance

- Level of consciousness:
- Orientation:
- Mood:
- Height:
- Weight:

Vital Signs

Temperature (°F/°C)	Pulse (beats/min)	Blood pressure (mm Hg)	Respiration (breath/min)

Head

Scalp	Face	Sinus	Nodes	Any other significant change

Eyes

Ocular movement	Pupils	Sclera	Cornea	Any other significant change

Ears

Tympanic membrane	Hearing		Any other significant change
	Weber's test	Rinne test	

Nose

Septum	Mucous membrane	Patency	Olfactory sense	Any other significant change

Mouth

Buccal mucosa	Gums/tongue	Palates and uvula	Tonsillar area	Voice breath	Any other significant change

Neck

Muscles	Trachea	Thyroid	Nodes	Vein distension	Any other significant change

Female Breast

Size and symmetry	Color	Areola	Nipples	Any other significant change

Thorax

Chest shape	Respiratory rate	Type of respiration	Thoracic expansion	Palpation	Percussion	Breath sounds

Cardiovascular System

Inspection	Palpation	Auscultation	Apical rate and rhythm	Any other significant change

Central and Peripheral Vessels

Peripheral pulses						
Brachial	Radial	Femoral	Popliteal	Dorsal pedal	Post tibial	Capillary refill

Abdomen

Inspection	Palpation	Auscultation	Percussion

Musculoskeletal System

Upper extremities	Lower extremities	Muscle strength	Joints	Range of motion	Gait	Spine

Nervous System

Pain	Orientation	Memory attention span	Level of consciousness Glasgow Coma Scale (GCS)	Cranial nerves	Deep tendon reflex	Gross and fine motor function	Temperature

Skin, Hair and Nails

Skin color	Any lesion on skin	Texture	Moisture	Temperature	Edema	Shape of nails

Genitalia and Rectal Examination

Inspection	Palpation (liver, spleen, kidney)	Ascites	Appendicitis	Pain	Any other significant change

Investigations

Date	Investigations done	Normal value	Patient value	Inference

Drug Study

S. No.	Drug trade name	Pharmacological name	Dose and frequency	Route	Action	Side effects and drug interaction	Nurses responsibility

Nursing Care Plan

Nursing assessment: Subjective and objective data	Nursing diagnosis	Goals	Nursing intervention		Rationale	Evaluation
			Planned	Implemented		

Nurses' Notes

Time	Medication	Diet/nutrition	Observation/ intervention/evaluation	Signature

Complications and Prognosis

Health Teaching

S. No.	Health education

Discharge Planning/Notes

Summary and Conclusions including Research Evidence

Bibliography

Evaluation Criteria for Nursing Care Plan – 2

S. No.	Contents	Maximum marks	Allotted marks
1.	Patient's History	02	
2.	Physical Examination	02	
3.	Investigations	01	
4.	Drug Study	02	
5.	Nursing Care Plan		
	• Assessment	02	
	• Nursing Diagnosis	02	
	• Goals	01	
	• Expected Outcome	01	
	• Nursing Intervention	03	
	• Rationale	01	
	• Evaluation	02	
6.	Nurses' Notes	03	
7.	Health Education	02	
8.	Bibliography	01	
	Total	**25**	

Remarks:

Signature of Student

Signature of Supervisor

NURSING CARE PLAN – 2

Patient's Identification Data

- Name:
- Age:
- Sex:
- Marital status:
- Hospital registration no.:
- Ward/bed no.:
- Address:
- Tel. no.:
- Religion:
- Education:
- Date of admission:
- Date of discharge:
- Diagnosis:
- Operation:
- Date of operation:
- Name of the doctor:
- Occupation:
- Monthly family income (₹):
- Nursing alert:
- Sensitivity/allergy/precaution:
- Weight:
- Height:

Chief Complaints with Duration

History of Present Illness

History of Past Medical Illness: Illness/medications/any restrictions

History of Past Surgical Illness: Illness/medications/any restrictions

Obstetrical History

No. of pregnancy	Year	Type of delivery	Gender of baby	Puerperium	Remarks

Family History

S. No.	Name of family member	Age and gender	Relationship with patient	Occupation	Health status/H/o significant illness	Health habits

Family Tree

Genogram key:

Female = ○

Male = □

Patient = Point to Patient ↗

Deceased = ■ or ●

( ) = Cause of death

⋮ = Adoption (vertical)

Consanguinity = □═○

Socioeconomic History

- Occupation and social relationship
- Monthly family income
- Health facility near home: Hospital/health center/any other: If any other (specify)

Transportation Facility

Yes/No

Housing

Type: Kutcha/Pucca
- Number of rooms
- Toilet: Indian/western/temporary/open
- Electricity: Yes/No
- Drinking water source: Tap/well/pond/river/hand/pump

Dietary History

Health Habits: Functional Health Pattern

- Health perception/health management:
- Nutritional/metabolic:
- Elimination:
- Activity/exercise:
- Sleep/rest:
- Self-perception/self-concept:
- Role relationship:
- Sexuality/reproductive:
- Coping/stress-tolerance:
- Value/belief:
- Other comments/data:

Physical Examination

General Appearance

- Level of consciousness:
- Orientation:
- Mood:
- Height:
- Weight:

Vital Signs

Temperature (°F/°C)	Pulse (beats/min)	Blood pressure (mm Hg)	Respiration (breath/min)

Head

Scalp	Face	Sinus	Nodes	Any other significant change

Eyes

Ocular movement	Pupils	Sclera	Cornea	Any other significant change

Ears

Tympanic membrane	Hearing		Any other significant change
	Weber's test	Rinne test	

Nose

Septum	Mucous membrane	Patency	Olfactory sense	Any other significant change

Mouth

Buccal mucosa	Gums/tongue	Palates and uvula	Tonsillar area	Voice breath	Any other significant change

Neck

Muscles	Trachea	Thyroid	Nodes	Vein distension	Any other significant change

Female Breast

Size and symmetry	Color	Areola	Nipples	Any other significant change

Thorax

Chest shape	Respiratory rate	Type of respiration	Thoracic expansion	Palpation	Percussion	Breath sounds

Cardiovascular System

Inspection	Palpation	Auscultation	Apical rate and rhythm	Any other significant change

Central and Peripheral Vessels

Peripheral pulses						
Brachial	Radial	Femoral	Popliteal	Dorsal pedal	Post tibial	Capillary refill

Abdomen

Inspection	Palpation	Auscultation	Percussion

Musculoskeletal System

Upper extremities	Lower extremities	Muscle strength	Joints	Range of motion	Gait	Spine

Nervous System

Pain	Orientation	Memory attention span	Level of consciousness Glasgow Coma Scale (GCS)	Cranial nerves	Deep tendon reflex	Gross and fine motor function	Temperature

Skin, Hair and Nails

Skin color	Any lesion on skin	Texture	Moisture	Temperature	Edema	Shape of nails

Genitalia and Rectal Examination

Inspection	Palpation (liver, spleen, kidney)	Ascites	Appendicitis	Pain	Any other significant change

Investigations

Date	Investigations done	Normal value	Patient value	Inference

Drug Study

S. No.	Drug trade name	Pharmacological name	Dose and frequency	Route	Action	Side effects and drug interaction	Nurses responsibility

Nursing Care Plan

Nursing assessment: Subjective and objective data	Nursing diagnosis	Goals	Nursing intervention		Rationale	Evaluation
			Planned	Implemented		

Nurses' Notes

Time	Medication	Diet/nutrition	Observation/ intervention/evaluation	Signature

Complications and Prognosis

Health Teaching

S. No.	Health education

Discharge Planning/Notes

Summary and Conclusions including Research Evidence

Bibliography

Evaluation Criteria for Nursing Care Plan – 3

S. No.	Contents	Maximum marks	Allotted marks
1.	Patient's History	02	
2.	Physical Examination	02	
3.	Investigations	01	
4.	Drug Study	02	
5.	Nursing Care Plan		
	◆ Assessment	02	
	◆ Nursing Diagnosis	02	
	◆ Goals	01	
	◆ Expected Outcome	01	
	◆ Nursing Intervention	03	
	◆ Rationale	01	
	◆ Evaluation	02	
6.	Nurses' Notes	03	
7.	Health Education	02	
8.	Bibliography	01	
	Total	**25**	

Remarks:

Signature of Student **Signature of Supervisor**

NURSING CARE PLAN – 3

Patient's Identification Data

- Name:
- Age:
- Sex:
- Marital status:
- Hospital registration no.:
- Ward/bed no.:
- Address:
- Tel. no.:
- Religion:
- Education:
- Date of admission:
- Date of discharge:
- Diagnosis:
- Operation:
- Date of operation:
- Name of the doctor:
- Occupation:
- Monthly family income (₹):
- Nursing alert:
- Sensitivity/allergy/precaution:
- Weight:
- Height:

Chief Complaints with Duration

History of Present Illness

History of Past Medical Illness: Illness/medications/any restrictions

History of Past Surgical Illness: Illness/medications/any restrictions

Obstetrical History

No. of pregnancy	Year	Type of delivery	Gender of baby	Puerperium	Remarks

Family History

S. No.	Name of family member	Age and gender	Relationship with patient	Occupation	Health status/H/o significant illness	Health habits

Family Tree

Genogram key:

Female = ○

Male = □

Patient = Point to Patient ↗

Deceased = ■ or ●

( ) = Cause of death

⋮ = Adoption (vertical)

Consanguinity = □═○

Socioeconomic History

- Occupation and social relationship
- Monthly family income
- Health facility near home: Hospital/health center/any other: If any other (specify)

Transportation Facility

Yes/No

Housing

Type: Kutcha/Pucca

- Number of rooms
- Toilet: Indian/western/temporary/open
- Electricity: Yes/No
- Drinking water source: Tap/well/pond/river/hand/pump

Dietary History

Health Habits: Functional Health Pattern

- Health perception/health management:
- Nutritional/metabolic:
- Elimination:
- Activity/exercise:
- Sleep/rest:
- Self-perception/self-concept:
- Role relationship:
- Sexuality/reproductive:
- Coping/stress-tolerance:
- Value/belief:
- Other comments/data:

Physical Examination

General Appearance

- Level of consciousness:
- Orientation:
- Mood:
- Height:
- Weight:

Vital Signs

Temperature (°F/°C)	Pulse (beats/min)	Blood pressure (mm Hg)	Respiration (breath/min)

Head

Scalp	Face	Sinus	Nodes	Any other significant change

Eyes

Ocular movement	Pupils	Sclera	Cornea	Any other significant change

Ears

Tympanic membrane	Hearing		Any other significant change
	Weber's test	Rinne test	

Nose

Septum	Mucous membrane	Patency	Olfactory sense	Any other significant change

Mouth

Buccal mucosa	Gums/tongue	Palates and uvula	Tonsillar area	Voice breath	Any other significant change

Neck

Muscles	Trachea	Thyroid	Nodes	Vein distension	Any other significant change

Female Breast

Size and symmetry	Color	Areola	Nipples	Any other significant change

Thorax

Chest shape	Respiratory rate	Type of respiration	Thoracic expansion	Palpation	Percussion	Breath sounds

Cardiovascular System

Inspection	Palpation	Auscultation	Apical rate and rhythm	Any other significant change

Central and Peripheral Vessels

Peripheral pulses						
Brachial	Radial	Femoral	Popliteal	Dorsal pedal	Post tibial	Capillary refill

Abdomen

Inspection	Palpation	Auscultation	Percussion

Musculoskeletal System

Upper extremities	Lower extremities	Muscle strength	Joints	Range of motion	Gait	Spine

Nervous System

Pain	Orientation	Memory attention span	Level of consciousness Glasgow Coma Scale (GCS)	Cranial nerves	Deep tendon reflex	Gross and fine motor function	Temperature

Skin, Hair and Nails

Skin color	Any lesion on skin	Texture	Moisture	Temperature	Edema	Shape of nails

Genitalia and Rectal Examination

Inspection	Palpation (liver, spleen, kidney)	Ascites	Appendicitis	Pain	Any other significant change

Investigations

Date	Investigations done	Normal value	Patient value	Inference

Drug Study

S. No.	Drug trade name	Pharmacological name	Dose and frequency	Route	Action	Side effects and drug interaction	Nurses responsibility

Nursing Care Plan

Nursing assessment: Subjective and objective data	Nursing diagnosis	Goals	Nursing intervention		Rationale	Evaluation
			Planned	Implemented		

Nurses' Notes

Time	Medication	Diet/nutrition	Observation/ intervention/evaluation	Signature

Complications and Prognosis

Health Teaching

S. No.	Health education

Discharge Planning/Notes

Summary and Conclusions including Research Evidence

Bibliography

Evaluation Criteria for Nursing Care Plan – 4

S. No.	Contents	Maximum marks	Allotted marks
1.	Patient's History	02	
2.	Physical Examination	02	
3.	Investigations	01	
4.	Drug Study	02	
5.	Nursing Care Plan		
	◆ Assessment	02	
	◆ Nursing Diagnosis	02	
	◆ Goals	01	
	◆ Expected Outcome	01	
	◆ Nursing Intervention	03	
	◆ Rationale	01	
	◆ Evaluation	02	
6.	Nurses' Notes	03	
7.	Health Education	02	
8.	Bibliography	01	
	Total	**25**	

Remarks:

Signature of Student **Signature of Supervisor**

NURSING CARE PLAN – 4

Patient's Identification Data

- Name:
- Age:
- Sex:
- Marital status:
- Hospital registration no.:
- Ward/bed no.:
- Address:
- Tel. no.:
- Religion:
- Education:
- Date of admission:
- Date of discharge:
- Diagnosis:
- Operation:
- Date of operation:
- Name of the doctor:
- Occupation:
- Monthly family income (₹):
- Nursing alert:
- Sensitivity/allergy/precaution:
- Weight:
- Height:

Chief Complaints with Duration

History of Present Illness

History of Past Medical Illness: Illness/medications/any restrictions

History of Past Surgical Illness: Illness/medications/any restrictions

Obstetrical History

No. of pregnancy	Year	Type of delivery	Gender of baby	Puerperium	Remarks

Family History

S. No.	Name of family member	Age and gender	Relationship with patient	Occupation	Health status/H/o significant illness	Health habits

Family Tree

Genogram key:

Female = ○

Male = □

Patient = Point to Patient ↗

Deceased = ■ or ●

( ) = Cause of death

⋮ = Adoption (vertical)

Consanguinity = □═○

Socioeconomic History

- Occupation and social relationship
- Monthly family income
- Health facility near home: Hospital/health center/any other: If any other (specify)

Transportation Facility

Yes/No

Housing

Type: Kutcha/Pucca

- Number of rooms
- Toilet: Indian/western/temporary/open
- Electricity: Yes/No
- Drinking water source: Tap/well/pond/river/hand/pump

Dietary History

Health Habits: Functional Health Pattern

- Health perception/health management:
- Nutritional/metabolic:
- Elimination:
- Activity/exercise:
- Sleep/rest:
- Self-perception/self-concept:
- Role relationship:
- Sexuality/reproductive:
- Coping/stress-tolerance:
- Value/belief:
- Other comments/data:

Physical Examination

General Appearance

- Level of consciousness:
- Oricntation:
- Mood:
- Height:
- Weight:

Vital Signs

Temperature (°F/°C)	Pulse (beats/min)	Blood pressure (mm Hg)	Respiration (breath/min)

Head

Scalp	Face	Sinus	Nodes	Any other significant change

Eyes

Ocular movement	Pupils	Sclera	Cornea	Any other significant change

Ears

Tympanic membrane	Hearing		Any other significant change
	Weber's test	Rinne test	

Nose

Septum	Mucous membrane	Patency	Olfactory sense	Any other significant change

Mouth

Buccal mucosa	Gums/tongue	Palates and uvula	Tonsillar area	Voice breath	Any other significant change

Neck

Muscles	Trachea	Thyroid	Nodes	Vein distension	Any other significant change

Female Breast

Size and symmetry	Color	Areola	Nipples	Any other significant change

Thorax

Chest shape	Respiratory rate	Type of respiration	Thoracic expansion	Palpation	Percussion	Breath sounds

Cardiovascular System

Inspection	Palpation	Auscultation	Apical rate and rhythm	Any other significant change

Central and Peripheral Vessels

Peripheral pulses						
Brachial	Radial	Femoral	Popliteal	Dorsal pedal	Post tibial	Capillary refill

Abdomen

Inspection	Palpation	Auscultation	Percussion

Musculoskeletal System

Upper extremities	Lower extremities	Muscle strength	Joints	Range of motion	Gait	Spine

Nervous System

Pain	Orientation	Memory attention span	Level of consciousness Glasgow Coma Scale (GCS)	Cranial nerves	Deep tendon reflex	Gross and fine motor function	Temperature

Skin, Hair and Nails

Skin color	Any lesion on skin	Texture	Moisture	Temperature	Edema	Shape of nails

Genitalia and Rectal Examination

Inspection	Palpation (liver, spleen, kidney)	Ascites	Appendicitis	Pain	Any other significant change

Investigations

Date	Investigations done	Normal value	Patient value	Inference

Drug Study

S. No.	Drug trade name	Pharmacological name	Dose and frequency	Route	Action	Side effects and drug interaction	Nurses responsibility

Nursing Care Plan

Nursing assessment: Subjective and objective data	Nursing diagnosis	Goals	Nursing intervention		Rationale	Evaluation
			Planned	Implemented		

Nurses' Notes

Time	Medication	Diet/nutrition	Observation/ intervention/evaluation	Signature

Complications and Prognosis

Health Teaching

S. No.	Health education

Discharge Planning/Notes

Summary and Conclusions including Research Evidence

Bibliography

Evaluation Criteria for Nursing Care Plan – 5

S. No.	Contents	Maximum marks	Allotted marks
1.	Patient's History	02	
2.	Physical Examination	02	
3.	Investigations	01	
4.	Drug Study	02	
5.	Nursing Care Plan		
	◆ Assessment	02	
	◆ Nursing Diagnosis	02	
	◆ Goals	01	
	◆ Expected Outcome	01	
	◆ Nursing Intervention	03	
	◆ Rationale	01	
	◆ Evaluation	02	
6.	Nurses' Notes	03	
7.	Health Education	02	
8.	Bibliography	01	
	Total	**25**	

Remarks:

Signature of Student

Signature of Supervisor

NURSING CARE PLAN – 5

Patient's Identification Data

- Name:
- Age:
- Sex:
- Marital status:
- Hospital registration no.:
- Ward/bed no.:
- Address:
- Tel. no.:
- Religion:
- Education:
- Date of admission:
- Date of discharge:
- Diagnosis:
- Operation:
- Date of operation:
- Name of the doctor:
- Occupation:
- Monthly family income (₹):
- Nursing alert:
- Sensitivity/allergy/precaution:
- Weight:
- Height:

Chief Complaints with Duration

History of Present Illness

History of Past Medical Illness: Illness/medications/any restrictions

History of Past Surgical Illness: Illness/medications/any restrictions

Obstetrical History

No. of pregnancy	Year	Type of delivery	Gender of baby	Puerperium	Remarks

Family History

S. No.	Name of family member	Age and gender	Relationship with patient	Occupation	Health status/H/o significant illness	Health habits

Family Tree

Genogram key:

Female = ○

Male = □

Patient = Point to Patient ↗

Deceased = ■ or ●

( ) = Cause of death

⋮ = Adoption (vertical)

Consanguinity = □═○

Socioeconomic History

- Occupation and social relationship
- Monthly family income
- Health facility near home: Hospital/health center/any other: If any other (specify)

Transportation Facility

Yes/No

Housing

Type: Kutcha/Pucca

- Number of rooms
- Toilet: Indian/western/temporary/open
- Electricity: Yes/No
- Drinking water source: Tap/well/pond/river/hand/pump

Dietary History

Health Habits: Functional Health Pattern

- Health perception/health management:
- Nutritional/metabolic:
- Elimination:
- Activity/exercise:
- Sleep/rest:
- Self-perception/self-concept:
- Role relationship:
- Sexuality/reproductive:
- Coping/stress-tolerance:
- Value/belief:
- Other comments/data:

Physical Examination

General Appearance

- Level of consciousness:
- Orientation:
- Mood:
- Height:
- Weight:

Vital Signs

Temperature (°F/°C)	Pulse (beats/min)	Blood pressure (mm Hg)	Respiration (breath/min)

Head

Scalp	Face	Sinus	Nodes	Any other significant change

Eyes

Ocular movement	Pupils	Sclera	Cornea	Any other significant change

Ears

Tympanic membrane	Hearing		Any other significant change
	Weber's test	Rinne test	

Nose

Septum	Mucous membrane	Patency	Olfactory sense	Any other significant change

Mouth

Buccal mucosa	Gums/tongue	Palates and uvula	Tonsillar area	Voice breath	Any other significant change

Neck

Muscles	Trachea	Thyroid	Nodes	Vein distension	Any other significant change

Female Breast

Size and symmetry	Color	Areola	Nipples	Any other significant change

Thorax

Chest shape	Respiratory rate	Type of respiration	Thoracic expansion	Palpation	Percussion	Breath sounds

Cardiovascular System

Inspection	Palpation	Auscultation	Apical rate and rhythm	Any other significant change

Central and Peripheral Vessels

Peripheral pulses						
Brachial	Radial	Femoral	Popliteal	Dorsal pedal	Post tibial	Capillary refill

Abdomen

Inspection	Palpation	Auscultation	Percussion

Musculoskeletal System

Upper extremities	Lower extremities	Muscle strength	Joints	Range of motion	Gait	Spine

Nervous System

Pain	Orientation	Memory attention span	Level of consciousness Glasgow Coma Scale (GCS)	Cranial nerves	Deep tendon reflex	Gross and fine motor function	Temperature

Skin, Hair and Nails

Skin color	Any lesion on skin	Texture	Moisture	Temperature	Edema	Shape of nails

Genitalia and Rectal Examination

Inspection	Palpation (liver, spleen, kidney)	Ascites	Appendicitis	Pain	Any other significant change

Investigations

Date	Investigations done	Normal value	Patient value	Inference

Drug Study

S. No.	Drug trade name	Pharmacological name	Dose and frequency	Route	Action	Side effects and drug interaction	Nurses responsibility

Nursing Care Plan

Nursing assessment: Subjective and objective data	Nursing diagnosis	Goals	Nursing intervention		Rationale	Evaluation
			Planned	Implemented		

Nurses' Notes

Time	Medication	Diet/nutrition	Observation/ intervention/evaluation	Signature

Complications and Prognosis

Health Teaching

S. No.	Health education

Discharge Planning/Notes

Summary and Conclusions including Research Evidence

Bibliography

Case Presentation

Evaluation Criteria for Nursing Case Study/Case Presentation – 1

S. No.	Contents	Maximum marks	Marks obtained
1.	Physical Arrangement	10	
2.	Assessment	10	
3.	Co-relation with Patient and Book	10	
4.	Medical, Surgical and Nursing Management	10	
5.	Drug Study	06	
6.	Nursing Care Plan	20	
7.	Nurses' Notes	05	
8.	Health Education	05	
9.	Use of AV Aids	05	
10.	Time Management	04	
11.	Group Participation/Discussion	05	
12.	Effectiveness/Styles of Presentation	05	
13.	References	05	
	Total	**100**	

Remarks:

Signature of Student **Signature of Supervisor**

NURSING CASE STUDY/CASE PRESENTATION – 1

Patient's Identification Data

- Name:
- Age:
- Sex:
- Marital status:
- Hospital registration no.:
- Ward/bed no.:
- Address:
- Tel. no.:
- Religion:
- Education:
- Date of admission:
- Date of discharge:
- Diagnosis:
- Operation:
- Date of operation:
- Name of the doctor:
- Occupation:
- Monthly family income (₹):
- Nursing alert:
- Sensitivity/allergy/precaution:
- Weight:
- Height:

Chief Complaints with Duration

History of Past Medical Illness: Illness/medications/any restrictions

History of Past Surgical Illness: Illness/medications/any restrictions

Obstetrical History

No. of pregnancy	Year	Type of delivery	Gender of baby	Puerperium	Remarks

Family History

S. No.	Name of family member	Age and gender	Relationship with patient	Occupation	Health status/H/o significant illness	Health habits

Family Tree

Genogram key:

Female = ○

Male = □

Patient = Point to Patient ↗

Deceased = ■ or ●

( ) = Cause of death

⋮ = Adoption (vertical)

Consanguinity = □═○

Socioeconomic History

- Occupation and social relationship
- Monthly family income
- Health facility near home: Hospital/health center/any other: If any other (specify)

Transportation Facility

Yes/No

Housing

Type: Kutcha/pucca
- Number of rooms
- Toilet: Indian/western/temporary/open
- Electricity: Yes/No
- Drinking water source: Tap/well/pond/river/hand/pump

Dietary History

Health Habits: Functional Health Pattern

- Health perception/health management:
- Nutritional/metabolic:
- Elimination:
- Activity/exercise:
- Sleep/rest:
- Self-perception/self-concept:
- Role relationship:
- Sexuality/reproductive:
- Coping/stress-tolerance:
- Value/belief:
- Other comments/data:

Physical Examination

General Appearance

- Level of consciousness:
- Orientation:
- Mood:
- Height:
- Weight:

Vital Signs

Temperature (°F/°C)	Pulse (beats/min)	Blood pressure (mm Hg)	Respiration (breath/min)

Head

Scalp	Face	Sinus	Nodes	Any other significant change

Eyes

Ocular movement	Pupils	Sclera	Cornea	Any other significant change

Ears

Tympanic membrane	Hearing		Any other significant change
	Weber's test	Rinne test	

Nose

Septum	Mucous membrane	Patency	Olfactory sense	Any other significant change

Mouth

Buccal mucosa	Gums/tongue	Palates and uvula	Tonsillar area	Voice breath	Any other significant change

Neck

Muscles	Trachea	Thyroid	Nodes	Vein distension	Any other significant change

Female Breast

Size and symmetry	Color	Areola	Nipples	Any other significant change

Thorax

Chest shape	Respiratory rate	Type of respiration	Thoracic expansion	Palpation	Percussion	Breath sounds

Cardiovascular System

Inspection	Palpation	Auscultation	Apical rate and rhythm	Any other significant change

Central and Peripheral Vessels

Peripheral pulses						
Brachial	Radial	Femoral	Popliteal	Dorsal pedal	Post tibial	Capillary refill

Abdomen

Inspection	Palpation	Auscultation	Percussion

Musculoskeletal System

Upper extremities	Lower extremities	Muscle strength	Joints	Range of motion	Gait	Spine

Nervous System

Pain	Orientation	Memory attention span	Level of consciousness (GCS)	Cranial nerves	Deep tendon reflex	Gross and fine motor function	Temperature

Skin, Hair and Nails

Skin color	Any lesion on skin	Texture	Moisture	Temperature	Edema	Shape of nails

Genitalia and Rectal Examination

Inspection	Palpation (liver, spleen, kidney)	Ascites	Appendicitis	Pain	Any other significant change

Investigations

Date	Investigations done	Normal value	Patient value	Inference

Drug Study

S. No.	Drug trade name	Pharmacological name	Dose and frequency	Route	Action	Side effects and drug interaction	Nurses responsibility

DISEASE CONDITION

Anatomy and Physiology Related to Disease Condition

Definition

Etiology and Risk Factors

Book picture	Patient picture

Pathophysiology

Book picture	Patient picture

Clinical Manifestations

Book picture	Patient picture

Diagnostic Evaluation

Book picture	Patient picture

Management (Medical and Surgical Management)

Book picture	Patient picture

Nursing Management

Book picture	Patient picture

Nursing Care Plan

Nursing assessment: Subjective and objective data	Nursing diagnosis	Goals	Nursing intervention		Rationale	Evaluation
			Planned	Implemented		

Nurses' Notes

Time	Medication	Diet/nutrition	Observation/ intervention/evaluation	Signature

Complications and Prognosis

S. No.	Complication	Prognosis

Health Teaching

S. No.	Health education

Discharge Planning/Notes

Summary and Conclusions including Research Evidence

Bibliography

Evaluation Criteria for Nursing Case Study/Case Presentation – 2

S. No.	Contents	Maximum marks	Marks obtained
1.	Physical Arrangement	10	
2.	Assessment	10	
3.	Co-relation with Patient and Book	10	
4.	Medical, Surgical and Nursing Management	10	
5.	Drug Study	06	
6.	Nursing Care Plan	20	
7.	Nurses' Notes	05	
8.	Health Education	05	
9.	Use of AV Aids	05	
10.	Time Management	04	
11.	Group Participation/Discussion	05	
12.	Effectiveness/Styles of Presentation	05	
13.	References	05	
	Total	**100**	

Remarks:

Signature of Student **Signature of Supervisor**

NURSING CASE STUDY/CASE PRESENTATION – 2

Patient's Identification Data

- Name:
- Age:
- Sex:
- Marital status:
- Hospital registration no.:
- Ward/bed no.:
- Address:
- Tel. no.:
- Religion:
- Education:
- Date of admission:
- Date of discharge:
- Diagnosis:
- Operation:
- Date of operation:
- Name of the doctor:
- Occupation:
- Monthly family income (₹):
- Nursing alert:
- Sensitivity/allergy/precaution:
- Weight:
- Height:

Chief Complaints with Duration

History of Past Medical Illness: Illness/medications/any restrictions

History of Past Surgical Illness: Illness/medications/any restrictions

Obstetrical History

No. of pregnancy	Year	Type of delivery	Gender of baby	Puerperium	Remarks

Family History

S. No.	Name of family member	Age and gender	Relationship with patient	Occupation	Health status/H/o significant illness	Health habits

Family Tree

Genogram key:

Female = ○

Male = □

Patient = Point to Patient

Deceased = ■ or ●

( ) = Cause of death

⋮ = Adoption (vertical)

Consanguinity = □═○

Socioeconomic History

- Occupation and social relationship
- Monthly family income
- Health facility near home: Hospital/health center/any other: If any other (specify)

Transportation Facility

Yes/No

Housing

Type: Kutcha/pucca
- Number of rooms
- Toilet: Indian/western/temporary/open
- Electricity: Yes/No
- Drinking water source: Tap/well/pond/river/hand/pump

Dietary History

Health Habits: Functional Health Pattern

- Health perception/health management:
- Nutritional/metabolic:
- Elimination:
- Activity/exercise:
- Sleep/rest:
- Self-perception/self-concept:
- Role relationship:
- Sexuality/reproductive:
- Coping/stress-tolerance:
- Value/belief:
- Other comments/data:

Physical Examination

General Appearance

- Level of consciousness:
- Orientation:
- Mood:
- Height:
- Weight:

Vital Signs

Temperature (°F/°C)	Pulse (beats/min)	Blood pressure (mm Hg)	Respiration (breath/min)

Head

Scalp	Face	Sinus	Nodes	Any other significant change

Eyes

Ocular movement	Pupils	Sclera	Cornea	Any other significant change

Ears

Tympanic membrane	Hearing		Any other significant change
	Weber's test	Rinne test	

Nose

Septum	Mucous membrane	Patency	Olfactory sense	Any other significant change

Mouth

Buccal mucosa	Gums/tongue	Palates and uvula	Tonsillar area	Voice breath	Any other significant change

Neck

Muscles	Trachea	Thyroid	Nodes	Vein distension	Any other significant change

Female Breast

Size and symmetry	Color	Areola	Nipples	Any other significant change

Thorax

Chest shape	Respiratory rate	Type of respiration	Thoracic expansion	Palpation	Percussion	Breath sounds

Cardiovascular System

Inspection	Palpation	Auscultation	Apical rate and rhythm	Any other significant change

Central and Peripheral Vessels

Peripheral pulses						
Brachial	Radial	Femoral	Popliteal	Dorsal pedal	Post tibial	Capillary refill

Abdomen

Inspection	Palpation	Auscultation	Percussion

Musculoskeletal System

Upper extremities	Lower extremities	Muscle strength	Joints	Range of motion	Gait	Spine

Nervous System

Pain	Orientation	Memory attention span	Level of consciousness (GCS)	Cranial nerves	Deep tendon reflex	Gross and fine motor function	Temperature

Skin, Hair and Nails

Skin color	Any lesion on skin	Texture	Moisture	Temperature	Edema	Shape of nails

Genitalia and Rectal Examination

Inspection	Palpation (liver, spleen, kidney)	Ascites	Appendicitis	Pain	Any other significant change

Investigations

Date	Investigations done	Normal value	Patient value	Inference

Drug Study

S. No.	Drug trade name	Pharmacological name	Dose and frequency	Route	Action	Side effects and drug interaction	Nurses responsibility

DISEASE CONDITION

Anatomy and Physiology Related to Disease Condition

Definition

Etiology and Risk Factors

Book picture	Patient picture

Pathophysiology

Book picture	Patient picture

Clinical Manifestations

Book picture	Patient picture

Diagnostic Evaluation

Book picture	Patient picture

Management (Medical and Surgical Management)

Book picture	Patient picture

Nursing Management

Book picture	Patient picture

Nursing Care Plan

Nursing assessment: Subjective and objective data	Nursing diagnosis	Goals	Nursing intervention		Rationale	Evaluation
			Planned	Implemented		

Nurses' Notes

Time	Medication	Diet/nutrition	Observation/ intervention/evaluation	Signature

Complications and Prognosis

S. No.	Complication	Prognosis

Health Teaching

S. No.	Health education

Discharge Planning/Notes

Summary and Conclusions including Research Evidence

Bibliography

Evaluation Criteria for Nursing Case Study/Case Presentation – 3

S. No.	Contents	Maximum marks	Marks obtained
1.	Physical Arrangement	10	
2.	Assessment	10	
3.	Co-relation with Patient and Book	10	
4.	Medical, Surgical and Nursing Management	10	
5.	Drug Study	06	
6.	Nursing Care Plan	20	
7.	Nurses' Notes	05	
8.	Health Education	05	
9.	Use of AV Aids	05	
10.	Time Management	04	
11.	Group Participation/Discussion	05	
12.	Effectiveness/Styles of Presentation	05	
13.	References	05	
	Total	**100**	

Remarks:

Signature of Student **Signature of Supervisor**

NURSING CASE STUDY/CASE PRESENTATION – 3

Patient's Identification Data

- Name:
- Age:
- Sex:
- Marital status:
- Hospital registration no.:
- Ward/bed no.:
- Address:
- Tel. no.:
- Religion:
- Education:
- Date of admission:
- Date of discharge:
- Diagnosis:
- Operation:
- Date of operation:
- Name of the doctor:
- Occupation:
- Monthly family income (₹):
- Nursing alert:
- Sensitivity/allergy/precaution:
- Weight:
- Height:

Chief Complaints with Duration

History of Past Medical Illness: Illness/medications/any restrictions

History of Past Surgical Illness: Illness/medications/any restrictions

Obstetrical History

No. of pregnancy	Year	Type of delivery	Gender of baby	Puerperium	Remarks

Family History

S. No.	Name of family member	Age and gender	Relationship with patient	Occupation	Health status/H/o significant illness	Health habits

Family Tree

Genogram key:

Female = ○

Male = □

Patient = Point to Patient ↗

Deceased = ■ or ●

( ) = Cause of death

⋮ = Adoption (vertical)

Consanguinity = □═○

Socioeconomic History

- Occupation and social relationship
- Monthly family income
- Health facility near home: Hospital/health center/any other: If any other (specify)

Transportation Facility

Yes/No

Housing

Type: Kutcha/pucca

- Number of rooms
- Toilet: Indian/western/temporary/open
- Electricity: Yes/No
- Drinking water source: Tap/well/pond/river/hand/pump

Dietary History

Health Habits: Functional Health Pattern

- Health perception/health management:
- Nutritional/metabolic:
- Elimination:
- Activity/exercise:
- Sleep/rest:
- Self-perception/self-concept:
- Role relationship:
- Sexuality/reproductive:
- Coping/stress-tolerance:
- Value/belief:
- Other comments/data:

Physical Examination

General Appearance

- Level of consciousness:
- Orientation:
- Mood:
- Height:
- Weight:

Vital Signs

Temperature (°F/°C)	Pulse (beats/min)	Blood pressure (mm Hg)	Respiration (breath/min)

Head

Scalp	Face	Sinus	Nodes	Any other significant change

Eyes

Ocular movement	Pupils	Sclera	Cornea	Any other significant change

Ears

Tympanic membrane	Hearing		Any other significant change
	Weber's test	Rinne test	

Nose

Septum	Mucous membrane	Patency	Olfactory sense	Any other significant change

Mouth

Buccal mucosa	Gums/tongue	Palates and uvula	Tonsillar area	Voice breath	Any other significant change

Neck

Muscles	Trachea	Thyroid	Nodes	Vein distension	Any other significant change

Female Breast

Size and symmetry	Color	Areola	Nipples	Any other significant change

Thorax

Chest shape	Respiratory rate	Type of respiration	Thoracic expansion	Palpation	Percussion	Breath sounds

Cardiovascular System

Inspection	Palpation	Auscultation	Apical rate and rhythm	Any other significant change

Central and Peripheral Vessels

Peripheral pulses						
Brachial	Radial	Femoral	Popliteal	Dorsal pedal	Post tibial	Capillary refill

Abdomen

Inspection	Palpation	Auscultation	Percussion

Musculoskeletal System

Upper extremities	Lower extremities	Muscle strength	Joints	Range of motion	Gait	Spine

Nervous System

Pain	Orientation	Memory attention span	Level of consciousness (GCS)	Cranial nerves	Deep tendon reflex	Gross and fine motor function	Temperature

Skin, Hair and Nails

Skin color	Any lesion on skin	Texture	Moisture	Temperature	Edema	Shape of nails

Genitalia and Rectal Examination

Inspection	Palpation (liver, spleen, kidney)	Ascites	Appendicitis	Pain	Any other significant change

Investigations

Date	Investigations done	Normal value	Patient value	Inference

Drug Study

S. No.	Drug trade name	Pharmacological name	Dose and frequency	Route	Action	Side effects and drug interaction	Nurses responsibility

DISEASE CONDITION

Anatomy and Physiology Related to Disease Condition

Definition

Etiology and Risk Factors

Book picture	Patient picture

Pathophysiology

Book picture	Patient picture

Clinical Manifestations

Book picture	Patient picture

Diagnostic Evaluation

Book picture	Patient picture

Management (Medical and Surgical Management)

Book picture	Patient picture

Nursing Management

Book picture	Patient picture

Nursing Care Plan

Nursing assessment: Subjective and objective data	Nursing diagnosis	Goals	Nursing intervention		Rationale	Evaluation
			Planned	Implemented		

Nurses' Notes

Time	Medication	Diet/nutrition	Observation/ intervention/evaluation	Signature

Complications and Prognosis

S. No.	Complication	Prognosis

Health Teaching

S. No.	Health education

Discharge Planning/Notes

Summary and Conclusions including Research Evidence

Bibliography

Evaluation Criteria for Nursing Case Study/Case Presentation – 4

S. No.	Contents	Maximum marks	Marks obtained
1.	Physical Arrangement	10	
2.	Assessment	10	
3.	Co-relation with Patient and Book	10	
4.	Medical, Surgical and Nursing Management	10	
5.	Drug Study	06	
6.	Nursing Care Plan	20	
7.	Nurses' Notes	05	
8.	Health Education	05	
9.	Use of AV Aids	05	
10.	Time Management	04	
11.	Group Participation/Discussion	05	
12.	Effectiveness/Styles of Presentation	05	
13.	References	05	
	Total	**100**	

Remarks:

Signature of Student **Signature of Supervisor**

NURSING CASE STUDY/CASE PRESENTATION – 4

Patient's Identification Data

- Name:
- Age:
- Sex:
- Marital status:
- Hospital registration no.:
- Ward/bed no.:
- Address:
- Tel. no.:
- Religion:
- Education:
- Date of admission:
- Date of discharge:
- Diagnosis:
- Operation:
- Date of operation:
- Name of the doctor:
- Occupation:
- Monthly family income (₹):
- Nursing alert:
- Sensitivity/allergy/precaution:
- Weight:
- Height:

Chief Complaints with Duration

History of Past Medical Illness: Illness/medications/any restrictions

History of Past Surgical Illness: Illness/medications/any restrictions

Obstetrical History

No. of pregnancy	Year	Type of delivery	Gender of baby	Puerperium	Remarks

Family History

S. No.	Name of family member	Age and gender	Relationship with patient	Occupation	Health status/H/o significant illness	Health habits

Family Tree

Genogram key:

Female = ○

Male = □

Patient = Point to Patient ↗

Deceased = ■ or ●

( ) = Cause of death

⋮ = Adoption (vertical)

Consanguinity = □═○

Socioeconomic History

- Occupation and social relationship
- Monthly family income
- Health facility near home: Hospital/health center/any other: If any other (specify)

Transportation Facility

Yes/No

Housing

Type: Kutcha/pucca

- Number of rooms
- Toilet: Indian/western/temporary/open
- Electricity: Yes/No
- Drinking water source: Tap/well/pond/river/hand/pump

Dietary History

Health Habits: Functional Health Pattern

- Health perception/health management:
- Nutritional/metabolic:
- Elimination:
- Activity/exercise:
- Sleep/rest:
- Self-perception/self-concept:
- Role relationship:
- Sexuality/reproductive:
- Coping/stress-tolerance:
- Value/belief:
- Other comments/data:

Physical Examination

General Appearance

- Level of consciousness:
- Orientation:
- Mood:
- Height:
- Weight:

Vital Signs

Temperature (°F/°C)	Pulse (beats/min)	Blood pressure (mm Hg)	Respiration (breath/min)

Head

Scalp	Face	Sinus	Nodes	Any other significant change

Eyes

Ocular movement	Pupils	Sclera	Cornea	Any other significant change

Ears

Tympanic membrane	Hearing		Any other significant change
	Weber's test	Rinne test	

Nose

Septum	Mucous membrane	Patency	Olfactory sense	Any other significant change

Mouth

Buccal mucosa	Gums/tongue	Palates and uvula	Tonsillar area	Voice breath	Any other significant change

Neck

Muscles	Trachea	Thyroid	Nodes	Vein distension	Any other significant change

Female Breast

Size and symmetry	Color	Areola	Nipples	Any other significant change

Thorax

Chest shape	Respiratory rate	Type of respiration	Thoracic expansion	Palpation	Percussion	Breath sounds

Cardiovascular System

Inspection	Palpation	Auscultation	Apical rate and rhythm	Any other significant change

Central and Peripheral Vessels

Peripheral pulses						
Brachial	Radial	Femoral	Popliteal	Dorsal pedal	Post tibial	Capillary refill

Abdomen

Inspection	Palpation	Auscultation	Percussion

Musculoskeletal System

Upper extremities	Lower extremities	Muscle strength	Joints	Range of motion	Gait	Spine

Nervous System

Pain	Orientation	Memory attention span	Level of consciousness (GCS)	Cranial nerves	Deep tendon reflex	Gross and fine motor function	Temperature

Skin, Hair and Nails

Skin color	Any lesion on skin	Texture	Moisture	Temperature	Edema	Shape of nails

Genitalia and Rectal Examination

Inspection	Palpation (liver, spleen, kidney)	Ascites	Appendicitis	Pain	Any other significant change

Investigations

Date	Investigations done	Normal value	Patient value	Inference

Drug Study

S. No.	Drug trade name	Pharmacological name	Dose and frequency	Route	Action	Side effects and drug interaction	Nurses responsibility

DISEASE CONDITION

Anatomy and Physiology Related to Disease Condition

Definition

Etiology and Risk Factors

Book picture	Patient picture

Pathophysiology

Book picture	Patient picture

Clinical Manifestations

Book picture	Patient picture

Diagnostic Evaluation

Book picture	Patient picture

Management (Medical and Surgical Management)

Book picture	Patient picture

Nursing Management

Book picture	Patient picture

Nursing Care Plan

Nursing assessment: Subjective and objective data	Nursing diagnosis	Goals	Nursing intervention		Rationale	Evaluation
			Planned	Implemented		

Nurses' Notes

Time	Medication	Diet/nutrition	Observation/ intervention/evaluation	Signature

Complications and Prognosis

S. No.	Complication	Prognosis

Health Teaching

S. No.	Health education

Discharge Planning/Notes

Summary and Conclusions including Research Evidence

Bibliography

Evaluation Criteria for Nursing Case Study/Case Presentation – 5

S. No.	Contents	Maximum marks	Marks obtained
1.	Physical Arrangement	10	
2.	Assessment	10	
3.	Co-relation with Patient and Book	10	
4.	Medical, Surgical and Nursing Management	10	
5.	Drug Study	06	
6.	Nursing Care Plan	20	
7.	Nurses' Notes	05	
8.	Health Education	05	
9.	Use of AV Aids	05	
10.	Time Management	04	
11.	Group Participation/Discussion	05	
12.	Effectiveness/Styles of Presentation	05	
13.	References	05	
	Total	**100**	

Remarks:

Signature of Student **Signature of Supervisor**

NURSING CASE STUDY/CASE PRESENTATION – 5

Patient's Identification Data

- Name:
- Age:
- Sex:
- Marital status:
- Hospital registration no.:
- Ward/bed no.:
- Address:
- Tel. no.:
- Religion:
- Education:
- Date of admission:
- Date of discharge:
- Diagnosis:
- Operation:
- Date of operation:
- Name of the doctor:
- Occupation:
- Monthly family income (₹):
- Nursing alert:
- Sensitivity/allergy/precaution:
- Weight:
- Height:

Chief Complaints with Duration

History of Past Medical Illness: Illness/medications/any restrictions

History of Past Surgical Illness: Illness/medications/any restrictions

Obstetrical History

No. of pregnancy	Year	Type of delivery	Gender of baby	Puerperium	Remarks

Family History

S. No.	Name of family member	Age and gender	Relationship with patient	Occupation	Health status/H/o significant illness	Health habits

Family Tree

Genogram key:

Female = ○

Male = □

Patient = Point to Patient ↗

Deceased = ■ or ●

( ) = Cause of death

⋮ = Adoption (vertical)

Consanguinity = □═○

Socioeconomic History

- Occupation and social relationship
- Monthly family income
- Health facility near home: Hospital/health center/any other: If any other (specify)

Transportation Facility

Yes/No

Housing

Type: Kutcha/pucca
- Number of rooms
- Toilet: Indian/western/temporary/open
- Electricity: Yes/No
- Drinking water source: Tap/well/pond/river/hand/pump

Dietary History

Health Habits: Functional Health Pattern

- Health perception/health management:
- Nutritional/metabolic:
- Elimination:
- Activity/exercise:
- Sleep/rest:
- Self-perception/self-concept:
- Role relationship:
- Sexuality/reproductive:
- Coping/stress-tolerance:
- Value/belief:
- Other comments/data:

Physical Examination

General Appearance

- Level of consciousness:
- Orientation:
- Mood:
- Height:
- Weight:

Vital Signs

Temperature (°F/°C)	Pulse (beats/min)	Blood pressure (mm Hg)	Respiration (breath/min)

Head

Scalp	Face	Sinus	Nodes	Any other significant change

Eyes

Ocular movement	Pupils	Sclera	Cornea	Any other significant change

Ears

Tympanic membrane	Hearing		Any other significant change
	Weber's test	Rinne test	

Nose

Septum	Mucous membrane	Patency	Olfactory sense	Any other significant change

Mouth

Buccal mucosa	Gums/tongue	Palates and uvula	Tonsillar area	Voice breath	Any other significant change

Neck

Muscles	Trachea	Thyroid	Nodes	Vein distension	Any other significant change

Female Breast

Size and symmetry	Color	Areola	Nipples	Any other significant change

Thorax

Chest shape	Respiratory rate	Type of respiration	Thoracic expansion	Palpation	Percussion	Breath sounds

Cardiovascular System

Inspection	Palpation	Auscultation	Apical rate and rhythm	Any other significant change

Central and Peripheral Vessels

Peripheral pulses						
Brachial	Radial	Femoral	Popliteal	Dorsal pedal	Post tibial	Capillary refill

Abdomen

Inspection	Palpation	Auscultation	Percussion

Musculoskeletal System

Upper extremities	Lower extremities	Muscle strength	Joints	Range of motion	Gait	Spine

Nervous System

Pain	Orientation	Memory attention span	Level of consciousness (GCS)	Cranial nerves	Deep tendon reflex	Gross and fine motor function	Temperature

Skin, Hair and Nails

Skin color	Any lesion on skin	Texture	Moisture	Temperature	Edema	Shape of nails

Genitalia and Rectal Examination

Inspection	Palpation (liver, spleen, kidney)	Ascites	Appendicitis	Pain	Any other significant change

Investigations

Date	Investigations done	Normal value	Patient value	Inference

Drug Study

S. No.	Drug trade name	Pharmacological name	Dose and frequency	Route	Action	Side effects and drug interaction	Nurses responsibility

DISEASE CONDITION

Anatomy and Physiology Related to Disease Condition

Definition

Etiology and Risk Factors

Book picture	Patient picture

Pathophysiology

Book picture	Patient picture

Clinical Manifestations

Book picture	Patient picture

Diagnostic Evaluation

Book picture	Patient picture

Management (Medical and Surgical Management)

Book picture	Patient picture

Nursing Management

Book picture	Patient picture

Nursing Care Plan

Nursing assessment: Subjective and objective data	Nursing diagnosis	Goals	Nursing intervention		Rationale	Evaluation
			Planned	Implemented		

Nurses' Notes

Time	Medication	Diet/nutrition	Observation/ intervention/evaluation	Signature

Complications and Prognosis

S. No.	Complication	Prognosis

Health Teaching

S. No.	Health education

Discharge Planning/Notes

Summary and Conclusions including Research Evidence

Bibliography

Drug Presentation

Evaluation Criteria for Drug Presentation – 1

S. No.	Contents	Maximum marks	Marks obtained
1.	Planning and Organization	05	
2.	Introduction and Classification	07	
3.	Factors Affecting Action of Drug	05	
4.	Trade and Pharmaceutical Names	03	
5.	Preparation, Strength and Dose	05	
6.	Indications and Contraindications	05	
7.	Action, Adverse Effect and Drug Interaction	08	
8.	Nursing Responsibilities	07	
9.	Conclusions	03	
10.	Bibliography	02	
	Total	**50**	

Remarks:

Signature of Student **Signature of Supervisor**

DRUG PRESENTATION – 1

Name of the Drug:

Ward:

Date:

Name of the Supervisor:

Introduction

Classification of Drug

Factors Affecting Action of Drug

Names of the Drug (Trade and Pharmaceutical Name)

Dose and Route

Dose	Route

Indications and Contraindications

Indications	Contraindications

Mechanism of Action

Adverse Effects and Drug Interactions

S. No.	Adverse drug effects	Drug interactions

Nursing Responsibilities

S. No.	Nursing responsibilities

Health Education to Patient or Family

S. No.	Health education

Conclusions

References

S. No.	References

EVALUATION CRITERIA FOR CARDIAC ASSESSMENT

S. No.	Contents	Marks	Marks obtained
1.	Inspection	10	
2.	Palpation	10	
3.	Auscultation	10	
4.	Documentation	10	
5.	Summary	10	
	Total	**50**	

Cardiovascular Assessment

Patient's Biodata

- Name:
- Age:
- Sex:
- Marital status:
- Hospital registration no.:
- Ward/bed no.:
- Address:
- Tel. no.:
- Religion:
- Education:
- Date of admission:
- Date of discharge:
- Diagnosis:
- Operation:
- Date of operation:
- Name of the doctor:
- Occupation:
- Monthly family income (₹):
- Nursing alert:
- Sensitivity/allergy/precaution:
- Weight:
- Height:

Performance criteria	Competency level			
Inspection	**Done correctly**	**Done with assistance**	**Not done**	**Comments**
◆ Begin the examination with the patient seated upright with the chest exposed				
◆ **Inspect the patient's face, lips, ears and scalp**				
◆ **Inspect the jugular veins for pulsation and distention** – With the patient sitting upright, adjust the lamp to the patient's neck – Patient's head is turned slightly away from the side you are examining – Look for the jugular veins for pulsation and distention				
◆ **If jugular vein pulsations are visible (measure the distention only on one side)** – Palpate the patient's radial pulse and determine whether the jugular vein pulsations coincide with the palpated radial pulse – Then have the patient lie at a 45° angle if the patient can tolerate this position – Place the first of the metric rulers vertically at the angle of Louis – Place the second metric ruler horizontally at a 90° angle to the first ruler – One end of this ruler should be at the angle of Louis and the other end in the jugular area on the lateral aspect of the neck – Raise the lateral portion of the horizontal ruler until it is at the top of the height of the distention and assess the height in centimeters of the elevation from the vertical ruler				
◆ **Inspect the carotid arteries** – With the patient still lying at a 45° angle – Using tangential lighting – Inspect the carotid arteries for pulsations				
◆ **Inspect the chest for pulsations** – Inspect the entire chest for pulsations – Observe the patient first in an upright position and then at a low-to mid Fowler's position – In particular, observe for pulsations, heaves or lifts over the five key landmarks				
Palpation				
◆ **Palpate the carotid pulses:** Note the rate, rhythm				

Performance criteria	Competency level			
Inspection	**Done correctly**	**Done with assistance**	**Not done**	**Comments**
• **Palpate the chest in the six areas for the apical impulse** – Remain on the client's right side and ask the client to remain supine – Use one or two finger pads to palpate the anterior chest for pulsation – Beginning with the aorta and proceed downward to the apex of the heart – Localize the apical impulse precisely by using pads of finger and asking the client to exhale and then hold it – Palpate the apical impulse in the mitral. You may ask the client to roll to the left side to better feel the impulse using the palmar surface of your hand				
Auscultation				
• **Auscultate for heart rate and rhythm** • **If you detect an irregular rhythm, auscultate for a pulse rate deficit by:** – Compare the apical pulse to a carotid pulse – Auscultate the apical pulse Simultaneously palpate a carotid pulse and compare the findings				
• **Auscultate to identify S1 and S2**				
• **Auscultate for extra heart sounds** – Roll the client towards the left side and listen with the bell at the apex for the presence of any extra heart sound – Aske the client to sit up and lean forward, and exhale – Use the bell of the stethoscope and listen at the aortic and pulmonic area				
Assessment of the peripheral vascular system				
• Place the patient in a sitting position on the examination table				
• Assessing blood pressure in both arms and legs				
Neck				
• Inspect the neck for carotid pulsations • Palpate the carotid pulses by using 2 or 3 fingers pads				

Performance criteria	Competency level			
Inspection	**Done correctly**	**Done with assistance**	**Not done**	**Comments**
Arms				
◆ **Assess the hands by** – Take the patient's hands in your hands – Inspect the color of skin and nail beds, the temperature and texture of the skin, and the presence of any lesions or swelling				
◆ **Observe for capillary refill in both hands**				
◆ **Palpate the radial pulse** – Repeat the procedure for another arm – Note the rate, rhythm, amplitude, and symmetry of the pulses				
◆ **Palpate both brachial pulses** – Repeat the procedure for another arm – Note the rate, rhythm, amplitude, and symmetry of the pulses				
◆ **Perform Allen's test** – If you suspect an obstruction or insufficiency of an artery in the arm – Allen's test may determine the patency of the radial and ulnar arteries – Ask the patient to place the hands on the knees with palms up – Compress the radial arteries of both wrists with your thumbs – Ask the patient to open and close his or her fist several times – While you are still compressing the radial arteries, ask the patient to open his or her hands				
Legs				
◆ **Inspect both legs** – Observe skin color, hair distribution, and any skin lesions – Skin color should match the skin tone of the rest of the body. Hair is normally present on the legs				
◆ **Compare the size of both legs** – Both legs should be symmetric in size. **If the legs are unequal** in size, measure the circumference of each leg at the widest point – It is important to measure each leg at the same point				

Performance criteria	Competency level			
Inspection	**Done correctly**	**Done with assistance**	**Not done**	**Comments**
◆ **Assess the legs for the presence of superficial veins** – With the patient in a sitting position and legs dangling from the examination table, inspect the legs – Now ask the patient to elevate the legs – The veins may appear as nodular bulges when the legs are in the dependent position, but any bulges should disappear when the legs are elevated – Palpate the veins for tenderness or inflammation (phlebitis)				
◆ **Palpate the legs bilaterally for temperature** using the dorsal surface of your hands				
◆ **Test for Homans' sign** – Assist the patient to a supine position – Flex the patient's knee about 5 degrees – Now sharply dorsiflex the patient's foot – Testing for Homans' sign – Ask whether the patient feels calf pain or not				
◆ **Palpate peripheral pulses bilaterally** femoral, popliteal, posterior tibial, dorsalis pedis				
◆ **Assess for arterial supply to the lower legs and feet (Buerger's test), if pulses in the legs are weak** – If you suspect an arterial deficiency, test for arterial supply to the lower extremities – Ask the patient to remain supine – Elevate the patient's legs 12 inches above the heart – Ask the patient to move the feet up and down at the ankles for 60 seconds to drain the venous blood – The skin will be blanched in color because only arterial blood is present – Now ask the patient to sit up and dangle the feet. Compare the color of both feet				
◆ **Check for edema of the legs:** If edema is present, you should grade it on a scale of 1+ (mild) to 4+ (severe)				
◆ Document your findings				

Signature of Student **Signature of Supervisor**

Evaluation Criteria for Drug Presentation – 2

S. No.	Contents	Maximum marks	Marks obtained
1.	Planning and Organization	05	
2.	Introduction and Classification	07	
3.	Factors Affecting Action of Drug	05	
4.	Trade and Pharmaceutical Names	03	
5.	Preparation, Strength and Dose	05	
6.	Indications and Contraindications	05	
7.	Action, Adverse Effect and Drug Interaction	08	
8.	Nursing Responsibilities	07	
9.	Conclusions	03	
10.	Bibliography	02	
	Total	**50**	

Remarks:

Signature of Student **Signature of Supervisor**

DRUG PRESENTATION – 2

Name of the Drug:

Ward:

Date:

Name of the Supervisor:

Introduction

Classification of Drug

Factors Affecting Action of Drug

Names of the Drug (Trade and Pharmaceutical Name)

Dose and Route

Dose	Route

Indications and Contraindications

Indications	Contraindications

Mechanism of Action

Adverse Effects and Drug Interactions

S. No.	Adverse drug effects	Drug interactions

Nursing Responsibilities

S. No.	Nursing responsibilities

Health Education to Patient or Family

S. No.	Health education

Conclusions

References

S. No.	References

Health Talk

Evaluation Criteria for Health Talk – 1

Name of the Student:

Topic:

Date and Time:

Group:

Ward:

Name of the Supervisor:

S. No.	Particulars	Total marks	Marks obtained
1.	Objectives: Clarity, Achievable General and Specific Objectives	3	
2.	Content: Comprehensive, Organized	8	
3.	AV Aids used: Suitable, Self-explanatory	5	
4.	Effectiveness of Presentation: Self-confidence, Appearance, Language, Manner, Group Participation	5	
5.	Time Plan: Timely Submission of Lesson Plan	2	
6.	References	2	
	Total	**25**	

Remarks:

Signature of Student

Signature of Supervisor

HEALTH TALK TO PATIENT AND FAMILY

Medical Disorders

Topic:

Name of the Ward:

Date and Time:

Group:

Name of the Student:

Name of the Supervisor:

General Objectives

Specific Objectives

Time	Specific objectives	Contents	Teaching/ learning activities	AV aids used	Evaluation

Time	Specific objectives	Contents	Teaching/ learning activities	AV aids used	Evaluation

Time	Specific objectives	Contents	Teaching/ learning activities	AV aids used	Evaluation

Time	Specific objectives	Contents	Teaching/ learning activities	AV aids used	Evaluation

Summary

References

S. No.	References

Evaluation Criteria for Health Talk – 2

Name of the Student:

Topic:

Date and Time:

Group:

Ward:

Name of the Supervisor:

S. No.	Particulars	Total marks	Marks obtained
1.	Objectives: Clarity, Achievable General and Specific Objectives	3	
2.	Content: Comprehensive, Organized	8	
3.	AV Aids used: Suitable, Self-explanatory	5	
4.	Effectiveness of Presentation: Self-confidence, Appearance, Language, Manner, Group Participation	5	
5.	Time Plan: Timely Submission of Lesson Plan	2	
6.	References	2	
	Total	**25**	

Remarks:

Signature of Student **Signature of Supervisor**

HEALTH TALK TO PATIENT AND FAMILY

Surgical Disorders

Topic:

Name of the Ward:

Date and Time:

Group:

Name of the Student:

Name of the Supervisor:

General Objectives

Specific Objectives

Time	Specific objectives	Contents	Teaching/ learning activities	AV aids used	Evaluation

Time	Specific objectives	Contents	Teaching/ learning activities	AV aids used	Evaluation

Time	Specific objectives	Contents	Teaching/ learning activities	AV aids used	Evaluation

Time	Specific objectives	Contents	Teaching/ learning activities	AV aids used	Evaluation

Summary

References

S. No.	References

Evaluation Criteria for Health Talk – 3

Name of the Student:

Topic:

Date and Time:

Group:

Ward:

Name of the Supervisor:

S. No.	Particulars	Total marks	Marks obtained
1.	Objectives: Clarity, Achievable General and Specific Objectives	3	
2.	Content: Comprehensive, Organized	8	
3.	AV Aids used: Suitable, Self-explanatory	5	
4.	Effectiveness of Presentation: Self-confidence, Appearance, Language, Manner, Group Participation	5	
5.	Time Plan: Timely Submission of Lesson Plan	2	
6.	References	2	
	Total	**25**	

Remarks:

Signature of Student

Signature of Supervisor

HEALTH TALK TO PATIENT AND FAMILY

Cardiac Disorders

Topic:

Name of the Ward:

Date and Time:

Group:

Name of the Student:

Name of the Supervisor:

General Objectives

Specific Objectives

Time	Specific objectives	Contents	Teaching/ learning activities	AV aids used	Evaluation

Time	Specific objectives	Contents	Teaching/ learning activities	AV aids used	Evaluation

Time	Specific objectives	Contents	Teaching/ learning activities	AV aids used	Evaluation

Time	Specific objectives	Contents	Teaching/ learning activities	AV aids used	Evaluation

Summary

References

S. No.	References

Evaluation Criteria for Health Talk – 4

Name of the Student:

Topic:

Date and Time:

Group:

Ward:

Name of the Supervisor:

S. No.	Particulars	Total marks	Marks obtained
1.	Objectives: Clarity, Achievable General and Specific Objectives	3	
2.	Content: Comprehensive, Organized	8	
3.	AV Aids used: Suitable, Self-explanatory	5	
4.	Effectiveness of Presentation: Self-confidence, Appearance, Language, Manner, Group Participation	5	
5.	Time Plan: Timely Submission of Lesson Plan	2	
6.	References	2	
	Total	**25**	

Remarks:

Signature of Student

Signature of Supervisor

HEALTH TALK TO PATIENT AND FAMILY

Musculoskeletal System Disorder

Topic:

Name of the Ward:

Date and Time:

Group:

Name of the Student:

Name of the Supervisor:

General Objectives

Specific Objectives

Time	Specific objectives	Contents	Teaching/ learning activities	AV aids used	Evaluation

Time	Specific objectives	Contents	Teaching/ learning activities	AV aids used	Evaluation

Time	Specific objectives	Contents	Teaching/ learning activities	AV aids used	Evaluation

Time	Specific objectives	Contents	Teaching/ learning activities	AV aids used	Evaluation

Summary

References

S. No.	References

Minor Operation Theater

Evaluation Criteria for Minor Operation Theater: Case – 1

Name of the Patient:

Diagnosis:

Name of the Surgery:

Name of the Surgeon:

S. No.	Particulars	Total marks	Marks obtained
1.	Identification Data	1	
2.	Preoperative Nursing Management	2	
3.	Intraoperative Procedure	2	
4.	Instrument used in Surgery	2	
5.	Immediate Postoperative Nursing Care	2	
6.	Summary	1	
	Total	**10**	

Remarks:

Signature of Student **Signature of Supervisor**

ASSIST AS A SCRUB NURSE IN MINOR OPERATION THEATER: CASE – 1

Name of the Patient: ....

Age: .... Gender: ....

IPD No.: .... Date of Admission: ....

Clinical Diagnosis:..

Name of Surgical Procedure: ....

Name of the Surgeon: ....

I. Preoperative Nursing Management

1. *Preoperative*

a. *Identification of Patient*

b. *Body Part Preparation*

c. *Preoperative Medications*

d. *Consent Form Signed by Patient/Family Member and Explained*

e. *Patient's Record and Report*

2. *Physical and Psychological Needs of Patient*

3. *Preoperative Health Teaching*

4. ***Vital Signs***

Temperature (°C/°F)	Pulse (beats/min.)	Respiration (breath/min.)	Blood pressure (mm Hg)	SpO_2 saturation	Level of pain

II. Intraoperative Nursing Management

1. ***Type of Anesthesia used:***
2. ***Specific Position of Patient:***
3. ***Instrument used***

4. ***Summary of Surgical Procedure***

5. ***Closure of Surgical Site***

6. ***Vital Signs***

Temperature (°C/°F)	Pulse (beats/min.)	Respiration (breath/min.)	Blood pressure (mm Hg)	SpO_2 saturation	Level of pain

III. Postoperative Nursing Management

1. ***Level of Consciousness:***
2. ***Condition of Surgical Site:***
3. ***Postoperative Medications***

4. *Special Instrument*

5. *Postoperative Teaching*

6. *Vital Signs*

Temperature (°C/°F)	Pulse (beats/min.)	Respiration (breath/min.)	Blood pressure (mm Hg)	SpO_2 saturation	Level of pain

Conclusions

Evaluation Criteria for Minor Operation Theater: Case – 2

Name of the Patient:

Diagnosis:

Name of the Surgery:

Name of the Surgeon:

S. No.	Particulars	Total marks	Marks obtained
1.	Identification Data	1	
2.	Preoperative Nursing Management	2	
3.	Intraoperative Procedure	2	
4.	Instrument used in Surgery	2	
5.	Immediate Postoperative Nursing Care	2	
6.	Summary	1	
	Total	**10**	

Remarks:

Signature of Student **Signature of Supervisor**

ASSIST AS A SCRUB NURSE IN MINOR OPERATION THEATER: CASE – 2

Name of the Patient: ....

Age: .... Gender: ....

IPD No.: .... Date of Admission: ....

Clinical Diagnosis: ....

Name of Surgical Procedure: ....

Name of the Surgeon: ....

I. Preoperative Nursing Management

1. *Preoperative*

a. *Identification of Patient*

b. *Body Part Preparation*

c. *Preoperative Medications*

d. *Consent Form Signed by Patient/Family Member and Explained*

e. *Patient's Record and Report*

2. *Physical and Psychological Needs of Patient*

3. *Preoperative Health Teaching*

4. *Vital Signs*

Temperature (°C/°F)	Pulse (beats/min.)	Respiration (breath/min.)	Blood pressure (mm Hg)	SpO_2 saturation	Level of pain

II. Intraoperative Nursing Management

1. *Type of Anesthesia used:*
2. *Specific Position of Patient:*
3. *Instrument used*

4. *Summary of Surgical Procedure*

5. ***Closure of Surgical Site***

6. ***Vital Signs***

Temperature (°C/°F)	Pulse (beats/min.)	Respiration (breath/min.)	Blood pressure (mm Hg)	SpO_2 saturation	Level of pain

III. Postoperative Nursing Management

1. ***Level of Consciousness:***
2. ***Condition of Surgical Site:***
3. ***Postoperative Medications***

4. *Special Instrument*

5. *Postoperative Teaching*

6. *Vital Signs*

Temperature (°C/°F)	Pulse (beats/min.)	Respiration (breath/min.)	Blood pressure (mm Hg)	SpO_2 saturation	Level of pain

Conclusions

Evaluation Criteria for Minor Operation Theater: Case – 3

Name of the Patient:

Diagnosis:

Name of the Surgery:

Name of the Surgeon:

S. No.	Particulars	Total marks	Marks obtained
1.	Identification Data	1	
2.	Preoperative Nursing Management	2	
3.	Intraoperative Procedure	2	
4.	Instrument used in Surgery	2	
5.	Immediate Postoperative Nursing Care	2	
6.	Summary	1	
	Total	**10**	

Remarks:

Signature of Student **Signature of Supervisor**

ASSIST AS A SCRUB NURSE IN MINOR OPERATION THEATER: CASE – 3

Name of the Patient: ....

Age: .... Gender: ....

IPD No.: .... Date of Admission: ....

Clinical Diagnosis:...

Name of Surgical Procedure: ....

Name of the Surgeon: ....

I. Preoperative Nursing Management

1. *Preoperative*

a. *Identification of Patient*

b. *Body Part Preparation*

c. *Preoperative Medications*

d. *Consent Form Signed by Patient/Family Member and Explained*

e. *Patient's Record and Report*

2. *Physical and Psychological Needs of Patient*

3. *Preoperative Health Teaching*

4. *Vital Signs*

Temperature (°C/°F)	Pulse (beats/min.)	Respiration (breath/min.)	Blood pressure (mm Hg)	SpO_2 saturation	Level of pain

II. Intraoperative Nursing Management

1. *Type of Anesthesia used:*

2. *Specific Position of Patient:*

3. *Instrument used*

4. *Summary of Surgical Procedure*

5. *Closure of Surgical Site*

6. *Vital Signs*

Temperature (°C/°F)	Pulse (beats/min.)	Respiration (breath/min.)	Blood pressure (mm Hg)	SpO_2 saturation	Level of pain

III. Postoperative Nursing Management

1. *Level of Consciousness:*

2. *Condition of Surgical Site:*

3. *Postoperative Medications*

4. ***Special Instrument***

5. ***Postoperative Teaching***

6. ***Vital Signs***

Temperature (°C/°F)	Pulse (beats/min.)	Respiration (breath/min.)	Blood pressure (mm Hg)	SpO_2 saturation	Level of pain

Conclusions

Evaluation Criteria for Minor Operation Theater: Case – 4

Name of the Patient:

Diagnosis:

Name of the Surgery:

Name of the Surgeon:

S. No.	Particulars	Total marks	Marks obtained
1.	Identification Data	1	
2.	Preoperative Nursing Management	2	
3.	Intraoperative Procedure	2	
4.	Instrument used in Surgery	2	
5.	Immediate Postoperative Nursing Care	2	
6.	Summary	1	
	Total	**10**	

Remarks:

Signature of Student

Signature of Supervisor

ASSIST AS A SCRUB NURSE IN MINOR OPERATION THEATER: CASE – 4

Name of the Patient: ....

Age: .... Gender: ....

IPD No.: .... Date of Admission: ....

Clinical Diagnosis: ....

Name of Surgical Procedure: ....

Name of the Surgeon: ....

I. Preoperative Nursing Management

1. *Preoperative*

a. *Identification of Patient*

b. *Body Part Preparation*

c. *Preoperative Medications*

d. *Consent Form Signed by Patient/Family Member and Explained*

e. *Patient's Record and Report*

2. *Physical and Psychological Needs of Patient*

3. *Preoperative Health Teaching*

4. *Vital Signs*

Temperature (°C/°F)	Pulse (beats/min.)	Respiration (breath/min.)	Blood pressure (mm Hg)	SpO_2 saturation	Level of pain

II. Intraoperative Nursing Management

1. *Type of Anesthesia used:*

2. *Specific Position of Patient:*

3. *Instrument used*

4. *Summary of Surgical Procedure*

5. ***Closure of Surgical Site***

6. ***Vital Signs***

Temperature (°C/°F)	Pulse (beats/min.)	Respiration (breath/min.)	Blood pressure (mm Hg)	SpO_2 saturation	Level of pain

III. Postoperative Nursing Management

1. ***Level of Consciousness:***
2. ***Condition of Surgical Site:***
3. ***Postoperative Medications***

4. *Special Instrument*

5. *Postoperative Teaching*

6. *Vital Signs*

Temperature (°C/°F)	Pulse (beats/min.)	Respiration (breath/min.)	Blood pressure (mm Hg)	SpO_2 saturation	Level of pain

Conclusions

Evaluation Criteria for Minor Operation Theater: Case – 5

Name of the Patient:

Diagnosis:

Name of the Surgery:

Name of the Surgeon:

S. No.	Particulars	Total marks	Marks obtained
1.	Identification Data	1	
2.	Preoperative Nursing Management	2	
3.	Intraoperative Procedure	2	
4.	Instrument used in Surgery	2	
5.	Immediate Postoperative Nursing Care	2	
6.	Summary	1	
	Total	**10**	

Remarks:

Signature of Student **Signature of Supervisor**

ASSIST AS A SCRUB NURSE IN MINOR OPERATION THEATER: CASE – 5

Name of the Patient: ....

Age: .... Gender: ....

IPD No.: .... Date of Admission: ....

Clinical Diagnosis:..

Name of Surgical Procedure: ....

Name of the Surgeon: ....

I. Preoperative Nursing Management

1. *Preoperative*

a. *Identification of Patient*

b. *Body Part Preparation*

c. *Preoperative Medications*

d. *Consent Form Signed by Patient/Family Member and Explained*

e. *Patient's Record and Report*

2. *Physical and Psychological Needs of Patient*

3. *Preoperative Health Teaching*

4. *Vital Signs*

Temperature (°C/°F)	Pulse (beats/min.)	Respiration (breath/min.)	Blood pressure (mm Hg)	SpO_2 saturation	Level of pain

II. Intraoperative Nursing Management

1. *Type of Anesthesia used:*

2. *Specific Position of Patient:*

3. *Instrument used*

4. *Summary of Surgical Procedure*

5. ***Closure of Surgical Site***

6. ***Vital Signs***

Temperature (°C/°F)	Pulse (beats/min.)	Respiration (breath/min.)	Blood pressure (mm Hg)	SpO_2 saturation	Level of pain

III. Postoperative Nursing Management

1. ***Level of Consciousness:***
2. ***Condition of Surgical Site:***
3. ***Postoperative Medications***

4. *Special Instrument*

5. *Postoperative Teaching*

6. *Vital Signs*

Temperature (°C/°F)	Pulse (beats/min.)	Respiration (breath/min.)	Blood pressure (mm Hg)	SpO_2 saturation	Level of pain

Conclusions

Major Operation Theater

Evaluation Criteria for Major Operation Theater: Case – 1

Name of the Patient:

Diagnosis:

Name of the Surgery:

Name of the Surgeon:

S. No.	Particulars	Total marks	Marks obtained
1.	Identification Data	1	
2.	Preoperative Nursing Management	2	
3.	Intraoperative Procedure	2	
4.	Instrument used in Surgery	2	
5.	Immediate Postoperative Nursing Care	2	
6.	Summary	1	
	Total	**10**	

Remarks:

Signature of Student **Signature of Supervisor**

ASSIST AS A SCRUB NURSE IN MAJOR OPERATION THEATER: CASE – 1

Name of the Patient: ....

Age: .... Gender: ....

IPD No.: .... Date of Admission: ....

Clinical Diagnosis:..

Name of Surgical Procedure: ....

Name of the Surgeon: ....

I. Preoperative Nursing Management

1. *Preoperative*

a. *Identification of Patient*

b. *Body Part Preparation*

c. *Preoperative Medications*

d. *Consent Form Signed by Patient/Family Member and Explained*

e. *Patient's Record and Report*

2. *Physical and Psychological Needs of Patient*

3. *Preoperative Health Teaching*

4. ***Vital Signs***

Temperature (°C/°F)	Pulse (beats/min.)	Respiration (breath/min.)	Blood pressure (mm Hg)	SpO_2 saturation	Level of pain

II. Intraoperative Nursing Management

1. ***Type of Anesthesia used:***
2. ***Specific Position of Patient:***
3. ***Instrument used***

4. ***Summary of Surgical Procedure***

5. ***Closure of Surgical Site***

6. ***Vital Signs***

Temperature (°C/°F)	Pulse (beats/min.)	Respiration (breath/min.)	Blood pressure (mm Hg)	SpO_2 saturation	Level of pain

III. Postoperative Nursing Management

1. ***Level of Consciousness:***

2. ***Condition of Surgical Site:***

3. ***Postoperative Medications***

4. *Special Instrument*

5. *Postoperative Teaching*

6. *Vital Signs*

Temperature (°C/°F)	Pulse (beats/min.)	Respiration (breath/min.)	Blood pressure (mm Hg)	SpO_2 saturation	Level of pain

Conclusions

Evaluation Criteria for Major Operation Theater: Case – 2

Name of the Patient:

Diagnosis:

Name of the Surgery:

Name of the Surgeon:

S. No.	Particulars	Total marks	Marks obtained
1.	Identification Data	1	
2.	Preoperative Nursing Management	2	
3.	Intraoperative Procedure	2	
4.	Instrument used in Surgery	2	
5.	Immediate Postoperative Nursing Care	2	
6.	Summary	1	
	Total	**10**	

Remarks:

Signature of Student **Signature of Supervisor**

ASSIST AS A SCRUB NURSE IN MAJOR OPERATION THEATER: CASE – 2

Name of the Patient: ....

Age: .... Gender: ....

IPD No.: .... Date of Admission: ....

Clinical Diagnosis: ....

Name of Surgical Procedure: ....

Name of the Surgeon: ....

I. Preoperative Nursing Management

1. *Preoperative*

a. *Identification of Patient*

b. *Body Part Preparation*

c. *Preoperative Medications*

d. *Consent Form Signed by Patient/Family Member and Explained*

e. *Patient's Record and Report*

2. *Physical and Psychological Needs of Patient*

3. *Preoperative Health Teaching*

4. ***Vital Signs***

Temperature (°C/°F)	Pulse (beats/min.)	Respiration (breath/min.)	Blood pressure (mm Hg)	SpO_2 saturation	Level of pain

II. Intraoperative Nursing Management

1. ***Type of Anesthesia used:***
2. ***Specific Position of Patient:***
3. ***Instrument used***

4. ***Summary of Surgical Procedure***

5. ***Closure of Surgical Site***

6. ***Vital Signs***

Temperature (°C/°F)	Pulse (beats/min.)	Respiration (breath/min.)	Blood pressure (mm Hg)	SpO_2 saturation	Level of pain

III. Postoperative Nursing Management

1. ***Level of Consciousness:***

2. ***Condition of Surgical Site:***

3. ***Postoperative Medications***

4. *Special Instrument*

5. *Postoperative Teaching*

6. ***Vital Signs***

Temperature (°C/°F)	Pulse (beats/min.)	Respiration (breath/min.)	Blood pressure (mm Hg)	SpO_2 saturation	Level of pain

Conclusions

Evaluation Criteria for Major Operation Theater: Case – 3

Name of the Patient:

Diagnosis:

Name of the Surgery:

Name of the Surgeon:

S. No.	Particulars	Total marks	Marks obtained
1.	Identification Data	1	
2.	Preoperative Nursing Management	2	
3.	Intraoperative Procedure	2	
4.	Instrument used in Surgery	2	
5.	Immediate Postoperative Nursing Care	2	
6.	Summary	1	
	Total	**10**	

Remarks:

Signature of Student **Signature of Supervisor**

ASSIST AS A SCRUB NURSE IN MAJOR OPERATION THEATER: CASE – 3

Name of the Patient: ....

Age: .... Gender: ....

IPD No.: .... Date of Admission: ....

Clinical Diagnosis: ....

Name of Surgical Procedure: ....

Name of the Surgeon: ....

I. Preoperative Nursing Management

1. *Preoperative*

a. *Identification of Patient*

b. *Body Part Preparation*

c. *Preoperative Medications*

d. *Consent Form Signed by Patient/Family Member and Explained*

e. *Patient's Record and Report*

2. *Physical and Psychological Needs of Patient*

3. *Preoperative Health Teaching*

4. ***Vital Signs***

Temperature (°C/°F)	Pulse (beats/min.)	Respiration (breath/min.)	Blood pressure (mm Hg)	SpO_2 saturation	Level of pain

II. Intraoperative Nursing Management

1. ***Type of Anesthesia used:***
2. ***Specific Position of Patient:***
3. ***Instrument used***

4. ***Summary of Surgical Procedure***

5. *Closure of Surgical Site*

6. *Vital Signs*

Temperature (°C/°F)	Pulse (beats/min.)	Respiration (breath/min.)	Blood pressure (mm Hg)	SpO_2 saturation	Level of pain

III. Postoperative Nursing Management

1. *Level of Consciousness:*

2. *Condition of Surgical Site:*

3. *Postoperative Medications*

4. *Special Instrument*

5. *Postoperative Teaching*

6. *Vital Signs*

Temperature (°C/°F)	Pulse (beats/min.)	Respiration (breath/min.)	Blood pressure (mm Hg)	SpO_2 saturation	Level of pain

Conclusions

Evaluation Criteria for Major Operation Theater: Case – 4

Name of the Patient:

Diagnosis:

Name of the Surgery:

Name of the Surgeon:

S. No.	Particulars	Total marks	Marks obtained
1.	Identification Data	1	
2.	Preoperative Nursing Management	2	
3.	Intraoperative Procedure	2	
4.	Instrument used in Surgery	2	
5.	Immediate Postoperative Nursing Care	2	
6.	Summary	1	
	Total	**10**	

Remarks:

Signature of Student **Signature of Supervisor**

ASSIST AS A SCRUB NURSE IN MAJOR OPERATION THEATER: CASE – 4

Name of the Patient: ....

Age: .... Gender: ....

IPD No.: .... Date of Admission: ....

Clinical Diagnosis: ....

Name of Surgical Procedure: ....

Name of the Surgeon: ....

I. Preoperative Nursing Management

1. *Preoperative*

a. *Identification of Patient*

b. *Body Part Preparation*

c. *Preoperative Medications*

d. *Consent Form Signed by Patient/Family Member and Explained*

e. *Patient's Record and Report*

2. *Physical and Psychological Needs of Patient*

3. *Preoperative Health Teaching*

4. *Vital Signs*

Temperature (°C/°F)	Pulse (beats/min.)	Respiration (breath/min.)	Blood pressure (mm Hg)	SpO_2 saturation	Level of pain

II. Intraoperative Nursing Management

1. *Type of Anesthesia used:*

2. *Specific Position of Patient:*

3. *Instrument used*

4. *Summary of Surgical Procedure*

5. ***Closure of Surgical Site***

6. ***Vital Signs***

Temperature (°C/°F)	Pulse (beats/min.)	Respiration (breath/min.)	Blood pressure (mm Hg)	SpO_2 saturation	Level of pain

III. Postoperative Nursing Management

1. ***Level of Consciousness:***
2. ***Condition of Surgical Site:***
3. ***Postoperative Medications***

4. *Special Instrument*

5. *Postoperative Teaching*

6. ***Vital Signs***

Temperature (°C/°F)	Pulse (beats/min.)	Respiration (breath/min.)	Blood pressure (mm Hg)	SpO_2 saturation	Level of pain

Conclusions

Evaluation Criteria for Major Operation Theater: Case – 5

Name of the Patient:

Diagnosis:

Name of the Surgery:

Name of the Surgeon:

S. No.	Particulars	Total marks	Marks obtained
1.	Identification Data	1	
2.	Preoperative Nursing Management	2	
3.	Intraoperative Procedure	2	
4.	Instrument used in Surgery	2	
5.	Immediate Postoperative Nursing Care	2	
6.	Summary	1	
	Total	**10**	

Remarks:

Signature of Student

Signature of Supervisor

ASSIST AS A SCRUB NURSE IN MAJOR OPERATION THEATER: CASE – 5

Name of the Patient: ....

Age: .... Gender: ....

IPD No.: .... Date of Admission: ....

Clinical Diagnosis:..

Name of Surgical Procedure: ....

Name of the Surgeon: ....

I. Preoperative Nursing Management

1. *Preoperative*

a. *Identification of Patient*

b. *Body Part Preparation*

c. *Preoperative Medications*

d. *Consent Form Signed by Patient/Family Member and Explained*

e. *Patient's Record and Report*

2. *Physical and Psychological Needs of Patient*

3. *Preoperative Health Teaching*

4. ***Vital Signs***

Temperature (°C/°F)	Pulse (beats/min.)	Respiration (breath/min.)	Blood pressure (mm Hg)	SpO_2 saturation	Level of pain

II. Intraoperative Nursing Management

1. ***Type of Anesthesia used:***
2. ***Specific Position of Patient:***
3. ***Instrument used***

4. ***Summary of Surgical Procedure***

5. *Closure of Surgical Site*

6. *Vital Signs*

Temperature (°C/°F)	Pulse (beats/min.)	Respiration (breath/min.)	Blood pressure (mm Hg)	SpO_2 saturation	Level of pain

III. Postoperative Nursing Management

1. *Level of Consciousness:*

2. *Condition of Surgical Site:*

3. *Postoperative Medications*

4. *Special Instrument*

5. *Postoperative Teaching*

6. *Vital Signs*

Temperature (°C/°F)	Pulse (beats/min.)	Respiration (breath/min.)	Blood pressure (mm Hg)	SpO_2 saturation	Level of pain

Conclusions

Positioning and Draping

Evaluation Criteria for Positioning and Draping: Case – 1

Name of the Patient:

Diagnosis:

Name of the Surgery:

Name of the Surgeon:

S. No.	Particulars	Total marks	Marks obtained
1.	Identification Data	1	
2.	Preoperative Nursing Management	2	
3.	Positioning Given to Patient	2	
4.	Steps used in Positioning	2	
5.	Immediate Postoperative Nursing Care	2	
6.	Summary	1	
	Total	**10**	

Remarks:

Signature of Student

Signature of Supervisor

POSITIONING AND DRAPING: CASE – 1

Name of the Patient: ....

Age: .... Gender: ....

IPD No: .... Date of Admission: ....

Clinical Diagnosis:...

Name of Surgical Procedure: ....

Name of the Surgeon: ....

I. Preoperative Nursing Management

1. *Preoperative*

a. *Identification of Patient*

b. *Body Part Preparation*

c. *Preoperative Medications*

d. *Consent Form Signed by Patient/Family Member and Explained*

e. *Patient's Record and Report*

2. ***Physical and Psychological Needs of Patient***

3. ***Preoperative Health Teaching***

4. *Vital Signs*

Temperature (°C/°F)	Pulse (beats/min.)	Respiration (breath/min.)	Blood pressure (mm Hg)	SpO_2 saturation	Level of pain

II. Positioning Given to Patient

III. Indications of Positioning Given to Patient

IV. Contraindications of Positioning Given to Patient

V. Postoperative Nursing Management

1. *Level of Consciousness*
2. *Condition of Surgical Site*
3. *Postoperative Medications*

4. *Special Instrument*

5. *Postoperative Teaching*

6. *Vital Signs*

Temperature (°C/°F)	Pulse (beats/min.)	Respiration (breath/min.)	Blood pressure (mm Hg)	SpO_2 saturation	Level of pain

Conclusions

Evaluation Criteria for Positioning and Draping: Case – 2

Name of the Patient:

Diagnosis:

Name of the Surgery:

Name of the Surgeon:

S. No.	Particulars	Total marks	Marks obtained
1.	Identification Data	1	
2.	Preoperative Nursing Management	2	
3.	Positioning Given to Patient	2	
4.	Steps used in Positioning	2	
5.	Immediate Postoperative Nursing Care	2	
6.	Summary	1	
	Total	**10**	

Remarks:

Signature of Student **Signature of Supervisor**

POSITIONING AND DRAPING: CASE – 2

Name of the Patient: ....

Age: .... Gender: ....

IPD No: .... Date of Admission: ....

Clinical Diagnosis:...

Name of Surgical Procedure: ....

Name of the Surgeon: ....

I. Preoperative Nursing Management

1. *Preoperative*

a. *Identification of Patient*

b. *Body Part Preparation*

c. *Preoperative Medications*

d. *Consent Form Signed by Patient/Family Member and Explained*

e. *Patient's Record and Report*

2. *Physical and Psychological Needs of Patient*

3. *Preoperative Health Teaching*

4. *Vital Signs*

Temperature (°C/°F)	Pulse (beats/min.)	Respiration (breath/min.)	Blood pressure (mm Hg)	SpO_2 saturation	Level of pain

II. Positioning Given to Patient

III. Indications of Positioning Given to Patient

IV. Contraindications of Positioning Given to Patient

V. Postoperative Nursing Management

1. ***Level of Consciousness***
2. ***Condition of Surgical Site***
3. ***Postoperative Medications***

4. ***Special Instrument***

5. ***Postoperative Teaching***

6. ***Vital Signs***

Temperature (°C/°F)	Pulse (beats/min.)	Respiration (breath/min.)	Blood pressure (mm Hg)	SpO_2 saturation	Level of pain

Conclusions

Evaluation Criteria for Positioning and Draping: Case – 3

Name of the Patient:

Diagnosis:

Name of the Surgery:

Name of the Surgeon:

S. No.	Particulars	Total marks	Marks obtained
1.	Identification Data	1	
2.	Preoperative Nursing Management	2	
3.	Positioning Given to Patient	2	
4.	Steps used in Positioning	2	
5.	Immediate Postoperative Nursing Care	2	
6.	Summary	1	
	Total	**10**	

Remarks:

Signature of Student **Signature of Supervisor**

POSITIONING AND DRAPING: CASE – 3

Name of the Patient: ....

Age: .... Gender: ....

IPD No: .... Date of Admission: ....

Clinical Diagnosis:...

Name of Surgical Procedure: ....

Name of the Surgeon: ....

I. Preoperative Nursing Management

1. *Preoperative*

a. *Identification of Patient*

b. *Body Part Preparation*

c. *Preoperative Medications*

d. *Consent Form Signed by Patient/Family Member and Explained*

e. *Patient's Record and Report*

2. *Physical and Psychological Needs of Patient*

3. *Preoperative Health Teaching*

4. ***Vital Signs***

Temperature (°C/°F)	Pulse (beats/min.)	Respiration (breath/min.)	Blood pressure (mm Hg)	SpO_2 saturation	Level of pain

II. Positioning Given to Patient

III. Indications of Positioning Given to Patient

IV. Contraindications of Positioning Given to Patient

V. Postoperative Nursing Management

1. ***Level of Consciousness***
2. ***Condition of Surgical Site***
3. ***Postoperative Medications***

4. ***Special Instrument***

5. *Postoperative Teaching*

6. *Vital Signs*

Temperature (°C/°F)	Pulse (beats/min.)	Respiration (breath/min.)	Blood pressure (mm Hg)	SpO_2 saturation	Level of pain

Conclusions

Evaluation Criteria for Positioning and Draping: Case – 4

Name of the Patient:

Diagnosis:

Name of the Surgery:

Name of the Surgeon:

S. No.	Particulars	Total marks	Marks obtained
1.	Identification Data	1	
2.	Preoperative Nursing Management	2	
3.	Positioning Given to Patient	2	
4.	Steps used in Positioning	2	
5.	Immediate Postoperative Nursing Care	2	
6.	Summary	1	
	Total	**10**	

Remarks:

Signature of Student

Signature of Supervisor

POSITIONING AND DRAPING: CASE – 4

Name of the Patient: ....

Age: .... Gender: ....

IPD No: .... Date of Admission: ....

Clinical Diagnosis:..

Name of Surgical Procedure: ....

Name of the Surgeon: ....

I. Preoperative Nursing Management

1. *Preoperative*

a. *Identification of Patient*

b. *Body Part Preparation*

c. *Preoperative Medications*

d. *Consent Form Signed by Patient/Family Member and Explained*

e. *Patient's Record and Report*

2. *Physical and Psychological Needs of Patient*

3. *Preoperative Health Teaching*

4. ***Vital Signs***

Temperature (°C/°F)	Pulse (beats/min.)	Respiration (breath/min.)	Blood pressure (mm Hg)	SpO_2 saturation	Level of pain

II. Positioning Given to Patient

III. Indications of Positioning Given to Patient

IV. Contraindications of Positioning Given to Patient

V. Postoperative Nursing Management

1. ***Level of Consciousness***
2. ***Condition of Surgical Site***
3. ***Postoperative Medications***

4. ***Special Instrument***

5. ***Postoperative Teaching***

6. ***Vital Signs***

Temperature (°C/°F)	Pulse (beats/min.)	Respiration (breath/min.)	Blood pressure (mm Hg)	SpO_2 saturation	Level of pain

Conclusions

Evaluation Criteria for Positioning and Draping: Case – 5

Name of the Patient:

Diagnosis:

Name of the Surgery:

Name of the Surgeon:

S. No.	Particulars	Total marks	Marks obtained
1.	Identification Data	1	
2.	Preoperative Nursing Management	2	
3.	Positioning Given to Patient	2	
4.	Steps used in Positioning	2	
5.	Immediate Postoperative Nursing Care	2	
6.	Summary	1	
	Total	**10**	

Remarks:

Signature of Student **Signature of Supervisor**

POSITIONING AND DRAPING: CASE – 5

Name of the Patient: ....

Age: .... Gender: ....

IPD No: .... Date of Admission: ....

Clinical Diagnosis: ....

Name of Surgical Procedure: ....

Name of the Surgeon: ....

I. Preoperative Nursing Management

1. *Preoperative*

a. *Identification of Patient*

b. *Body Part Preparation*

c. *Preoperative Medications*

d. *Consent Form Signed by Patient/Family Member and Explained*

e. *Patient's Record and Report*

2. *Physical and Psychological Needs of Patient*

3. *Preoperative Health Teaching*

4. *Vital Signs*

Temperature (°C/°F)	Pulse (beats/min.)	Respiration (breath/min.)	Blood pressure (mm Hg)	SpO_2 saturation	Level of pain

II. Positioning Given to Patient

III. Indications of Positioning Given to Patient

IV. Contraindications of Positioning Given to Patient

V. Postoperative Nursing Management

1. ***Level of Consciousness***
2. ***Condition of Surgical Site***
3. ***Postoperative Medications***

4. ***Special Instrument***

5. *Postoperative Teaching*

6. *Vital Signs*

Temperature (°C/°F)	Pulse (beats/min.)	Respiration (breath/min.)	Blood pressure (mm Hg)	SpO_2 saturation	Level of pain

Conclusions

Assist as Circulatory Nurse

Evaluation Criteria for Assist as Circulatory Nurse: Case – 1

Name of the Patient:

Diagnosis:

Name of the Surgery:

Name of the Surgeon:

S. No.	Particulars	Total Marks	Marks Obtained
1.	Identification Data	1	
2.	Preoperative Nursing Management	2	
3.	Instrument used in Surgery	2	
4.	Immediate Postoperative Nursing Care	2	
5.	Summary	1	
	Total	**8**	

Remarks:

Signature of Student **Signature of Supervisor**

ASSIST AS CIRCULATORY NURSE: CASE – 1

Name of the Patient: ....

Age: .... Gender: ....

IPD No: .... Date of Admission: ....

Clinical Diagnosis:..

Name of Surgical Procedure: ....

Name of the Surgeon: ....

I. Preoperative Nursing Management

1. *Preoperative*

a. *Identification of Patient*

b. *Body Part Preparation*

c. *Preoperative Medications*

d. *Consent Form Signed by Patient/Family Member and Explained*

e. *Patient's Record and Report*

2. *Physical and Psychological Needs of Patient*

3. *Preoperative Health Teaching*

4. *Vital Signs*

Temperature (°C/°F)	Pulse (beats/min.)	Respiration (breath/min.)	Blood pressure (mm Hg)	SpO_2 saturation	Level of pain

II. Postoperative Nursing Management

1. *Level of Consciousness*
2. *Condition of Surgical Site*
3. *Postoperative Medications*

4. *Special Instrument*

5. *Postoperative Teaching*

6. *Vital Signs*

Temperature (°C/°F)	Pulse (beats/min.)	Respiration (breath/min.)	Blood pressure (mm Hg)	SpO_2 saturation	Level of pain

Conclusions

Evaluation Criteria for Assist as Circulatory Nurse: Case – 2

Name of the Patient:

Diagnosis:

Name of the Surgery:

Name of the Surgeon:

S. No.	Particulars	Total Marks	Marks Obtained
1.	Identification Data	1	
2.	Preoperative Nursing Management	2	
3.	Instrument used in Surgery	2	
4.	Immediate Postoperative Nursing Care	2	
5.	Summary	1	
	Total	**8**	

Remarks:

Signature of Student **Signature of Supervisor**

ASSIST AS CIRCULATORY NURSE: CASE – 2

Name of the Patient: ....

Age: .... Gender: ....

IPD No: .... Date of Admission: ....

Clinical Diagnosis: ....

Name of Surgical Procedure: ....

Name of the Surgeon: ....

I. Preoperative Nursing Management

1. *Preoperative*

a. *Identification of Patient*

b. *Body Part Preparation*

c. *Preoperative Medications*

d. *Consent Form Signed by Patient/Family Member and Explained*

e. *Patient's Record and Report*

2. *Physical and Psychological Needs of Patient*

3. *Preoperative Health Teaching*

4. *Vital Signs*

Temperature (°C/°F)	Pulse (beats/min.)	Respiration (breath/min.)	Blood pressure (mm Hg)	SpO_2 saturation	Level of pain

II. Postoperative Nursing Management

1. *Level of Consciousness*

2. *Condition of Surgical Site*

3. *Postoperative Medications*

4. *Special Instrument*

5. *Postoperative Teaching*

6. ***Vital Signs***

Temperature (°C/°F)	Pulse (beats/min.)	Respiration (breath/min.)	Blood pressure (mm Hg)	SpO_2 saturation	Level of pain

Conclusions

Evaluation Criteria for Assist as Circulatory Nurse: Case – 3

Name of the Patient:

Diagnosis:

Name of the Surgery:

Name of the Surgeon:

S. No.	Particulars	Total Marks	Marks Obtained
1.	Identification Data	1	
2.	Preoperative Nursing Management	2	
3.	Instrument used in Surgery	2	
4.	Immediate Postoperative Nursing Care	2	
5.	Summary	1	
	Total	**8**	

Remarks:

Signature of Student

Signature of Supervisor

ASSIST AS CIRCULATORY NURSE: CASE – 3

Name of the Patient: ....

Age: .... Gender: ....

IPD No: .... Date of Admission: ....

Clinical Diagnosis:..

Name of Surgical Procedure: ....

Name of the Surgeon: ....

I. Preoperative Nursing Management

1. *Preoperative*

a. *Identification of Patient*

b. *Body Part Preparation*

c. *Preoperative Medications*

d. *Consent Form Signed by Patient/Family Member and Explained*

e. *Patient's Record and Report*

2. *Physical and Psychological Needs of Patient*

3. *Preoperative Health Teaching*

4. *Vital Signs*

Temperature (°C/°F)	Pulse (beats/min.)	Respiration (breath/min.)	Blood pressure (mm Hg)	SpO_2 saturation	Level of pain

II. Postoperative Nursing Management

1. *Level of Consciousness*
2. *Condition of Surgical Site*
3. *Postoperative Medications*

4. *Special Instrument*

5. *Postoperative Teaching*

6. ***Vital Signs***

Temperature (°C/°F)	Pulse (beats/min.)	Respiration (breath/min.)	Blood pressure (mm Hg)	SpO_2 saturation	Level of pain

Conclusions

Evaluation Criteria for Assist as Circulatory Nurse: Case – 4

Name of the Patient:

Diagnosis:

Name of the Surgery:

Name of the Surgeon:

S. No.	Particulars	Total Marks	Marks Obtained
1.	Identification Data	1	
2.	Preoperative Nursing Management	2	
3.	Instrument used in Surgery	2	
4.	Immediate Postoperative Nursing Care	2	
5.	Summary	1	
	Total	**8**	

Remarks:

Signature of Student

Signature of Supervisor

ASSIST AS CIRCULATORY NURSE: CASE – 4

Name of the Patient: ....

Age: .... Gender: ....

IPD No: .... Date of Admission: ....

Clinical Diagnosis:...

Name of Surgical Procedure: ....

Name of the Surgeon: ....

I. Preoperative Nursing Management

1. *Preoperative*

a. *Identification of Patient*

b. *Body Part Preparation*

c. *Preoperative Medications*

d. *Consent Form Signed by Patient/Family Member and Explained*

e. *Patient's Record and Report*

2. ***Physical and Psychological Needs of Patient***

3. ***Preoperative Health Teaching***

4. ***Vital Signs***

Temperature (°C/°F)	Pulse (beats/min.)	Respiration (breath/min.)	Blood pressure (mm Hg)	SpO_2 saturation	Level of pain

II. Postoperative Nursing Management

1. ***Level of Consciousness***
2. ***Condition of Surgical Site***
3. ***Postoperative Medications***

4. ***Special Instrument***

5. ***Postoperative Teaching***

6. ***Vital Signs***

Temperature (°C/°F)	Pulse (beats/min.)	Respiration (breath/min.)	Blood pressure (mm Hg)	SpO_2 saturation	Level of pain

Conclusions